SHIATSU

Chris Jarmey is a state registered physiotherapist who has been studying, practising
and subsequently teaching Shiatsu since
1970. In 1985 he founded the European
Shiatsu School, which teaches Shiatsu up to
practitioner level and has branches throughout Britain and Europe. He is the Principal of
the ESS and regularly sits on the Core Group
and Examining Board of the Shiatsu Society.

IN THE SAME SERIES:

Principles of Aromatherapy
Cathy Hopkins

Principles of Buddhism
Kulananda

Principles of Chinese Medicine
Angela Hicks

Principles of Colonic Irrigation
Jillie Collings

Principles of the Enneagram
Karen Webb

Principles of Hypnotherapy
Vera Peiffer

Principles of NLP
Joseph O'Connor and Ian McDermott

Principles of Nutritional Therapy
Linda Lazarides

Principles of Paganism
Vivianne Crowley

Principles of Reflexology
Nicola Hall

Principles of Self-healing
David Lawson

Principles of Stress Management
Vera Peiffer

Principles of Tarot
Evelyn and Terry Donaldson

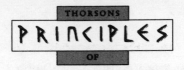

THORSONS
PRINCIPLES OF

SHIATSU

CHRIS JARMEY

Thorsons
An Imprint of HarperCollins*Publishers*

Thorsons
An Imprint of HarperCollins*Publishers*
77–85 Fulham Palace Road,
Hammersmith, London W6 8JB
1160 Battery Street,
San Francisco, California 94111–1213

Originally published as
*Thorsons Introductory Guide to Shiatsu*1992
This edition published by Thorsons 1996

1 3 5 7 9 10 8 6 4 2

© Chris Jarmey 1992, 1996

Chris Jarmey asserts the moral right to
be identified as the author of this work

A catalogue record for this book
is available from the British Library

ISBN 0 7225 3362 4

Printed in Great Britain by
Caledonian International Book Manufacturing Ltd, Glasgow

CONTENTS

Introduction   vii

1   How is Shiatsu Applied?   1
2   The Basics of Oriental Medicine   8
3   What to Expect When Attending a Treatment   72
4   Treating Specific Ailments   93
5   Adjuncts to Shiatsu Theory and Practice   160
6   Case Histories and Other Applications   164

Resources   176
Index   178

INTRODUCTION

WHAT IS SHIATSU?

S hiatsu is a Japanese word which literally translated means 'finger pressure'. This implies that pressure given to a body using the fingers is the predominant method of applying Shiatsu to stimulate a healing response. However, Shiatsu is much more than that. Its techniques involve the use not only of fingers, but also thumbs, palms, knees, forearms, elbows and feet. Moreover, since it is given on the floor rather than on a couch, it gives considerable attention to the correct use of body positioning and gravity to deliver its wide range of techniques.

At a level of first aid and stress relief it can be administered to good effect by the lay person with very little experience, who will also find it of great value in helping close friends and associates to relax and feel more 'balanced'. However, the full potential of Shiatsu is only realized after certain qualities have been developed within the giver. These qualities are:

- The ability to remain relaxed and comfortable irrespective of which technique is employed at any given time.

- The ability to detect subtle changes in a person's vitality through the medium of touch.

- The ability to assess a person's level of health or disease through the development of greater empathy and the understanding of Oriental Medicine.

Shiatsu can therefore be classified as a physical therapy applied at floor level with minimum physical effort by the therapist, and which uses Oriental Medicine as its theoretical framework. It generally takes at least three years of committed study and practice to reach a professional standard of competence, but even after a few days of tuition, its most fundamental principles can be applied at a domestic level.

Shiatsu is about communicating with others and offering them your support through touch, as much as it is about physical therapy. It requires feeling, both in a tactile sense and at an emotional level, and it also requires thinking.

Beyond its role in the healing of others, Shiatsu is also a tremendous method of self-development. It has the effect of focusing the mind and grounding both body and mind in much the same way as the practice of Tai Ji Quan (sometimes spelt Tai Chi Chuan), Yoga and various forms of meditation. For this reason it heals, strengthens and develops both giver and the recipient. Therefore, if given conscientiously, everything about Shiatsu is positive for everyone involved. Nobody loses and everybody gains!

WHAT IS THE PURPOSE OF THIS BOOK?

This book is written for those who are generally curious about Shiatsu and for those of you who are considering getting some Shiatsu treatment. Beginner Shiatsu students will also find much useful information within these pages. I intend to give you an idea of the full potential of Shiatsu, and how it can be of value to you personally. I will show you what you can expect to gain from a series of treatments, plus indicate some simple self-help methods which you can administer to yourself or to your friends. If you read this book carefully, you should grasp many of the fundamental principles of traditional Oriental Medicine, which forms the theoretical basis of Shiatsu, Acupuncture and Chinese Herbal Medicine.

There is a list of book titles on page 177 for those of you who, after reading this book, wish to learn more.

THE HISTORY OF SHIATSU

Although the word Shiatsu was not coined until the early twentieth century, the origins of Shiatsu lie firmly within the roots of Traditional Oriental Medicine. Specifically, it can be traced to China around 530 BC, when a system of exercises for health and sensory control known as Tao-Yinn was introduced. These incorporated a system of self-massage and self-applied pressure point therapy for promoting detoxification and rejuvenation. Tao-Yinn soon became an integral part of the health practices and was gradually exported, along with the other Chinese healing arts, through south-east Asia and Korea.

By the tenth century AD, Chinese Medicine had been introduced into Japan, from which time an amalgam of vibrational palm healing, acupressure and massage, known collectively as Anma, would have been combined with Tao-Yinn (Do-In) to loosely resemble present-day Shiatsu.

Around three hundred years ago, during the Edo era in Japan, doctors were required to study Anma as a means of familiarizing themselves with the human structure, energy Channels and pressure points, so that they could accurately diagnose and treat with whatever means they thought appropriate; namely acupuncture, herbal medicine or bodywork. Gradually, however, Anma was reduced to treating simple

x muscular tensions until by the twentieth century it became licensed only to promote pleasure and comfort.

However, there still existed many Anma therapists who based their work on the original theory, and who coined the name Shiatsu in order to avoid the restrictive regulations applied to Anma. Shiatsu was eventually recognized as a legitimate form of therapy by the Japanese government in the mid-1950s.

Nowadays the official definition given by the Japanese Ministry of Health and Welfare states:

'Shiatsu therapy is a form of manipulation administered by the thumbs, fingers and palms, without the use of any instrument, mechanical or otherwise, to apply pressure to the human skin, to correct internal malfunctioning, promote and maintain health and treat specific diseases.'

Shiatsu did not become widely known in Europe and the United States until the 1970s, although it has been practised by a few Japanese and Occidentals in the West since its conception.

HOW IS SHIATSU APPLIED?

THE SHIATSU ENVIRONMENT

One of the attractions of Shiatsu is that it needs no special equipment. All that is required is a floor area large enough for you to lie down upon, plus space for the practitioner to crawl around you. Unless you happen to be lying on a very thick carpet, it is more comfortable to have a padded but firm mat underneath you. A futon of two to three layers is ideal, preferably wide enough to allow the practitioner's knees some cushioning. A clean sheet on top of the futon, at least large enough for your face, helps maintain a sense of freshness and professionalism. However, even without these things Shiatsu can still be applied with you sitting on a cushion or chair. This all adds up to a very versatile form of bodywork.

You are not even required to undress for Shiatsu. In fact it is *better* done through clothing, as working on the skin stimulates too many superficial sensory nerves, thus distracting you from experiencing deeper sensations. The practitioner can also feel for deeper levels of imbalance in your body when the sensation of skin to skin contact is removed. Obviously, nobody will feel anything through an anorak and jumper. The ideal is a single layer of cotton garments. Cotton and other natural fibres are neutral to the touch. Nylon and most other synthetic fibres are full of static electricity and are particularly distractive of deep tactile sensations.

All these factors enable you to receive Shiatsu just about anywhere; in the office, in the garden, on the train or on the plane. However, I am sure most of you would prefer Shiatsu in a nice quiet, simply but tastefully decorated room. Fortunately, most Shiatsu 'studios' are like that.

THE 'TOOLS' OF SHIATSU

Various parts of the practitioner's limbs constitute the 'tools' of Shiatsu. The primary tools are the palms, thumbs and fingers. Tools of secondary importance, but nevertheless very useful, are the forearms, elbows, knees and feet. Your Shiatsu therapist will employ some or all of these tools throughout the course of a single treatment.

The palms and fingertips are used at the beginning of a treatment to feel for areas in your body in need of decongesting, loosening up, calming down, or strengthening. The fingertips in particular are extremely rich in sensory nerve endings and as such, are especially sensitive. An experienced Shiatsu therapist will have developed this sensitivity to its maximum potential. This gives him or her the ability to 'feel out' subtle imbalances in your blood circulation, muscle tone and energy flow. With an accompanying knowledge of Oriental Medicine and diagnosis, the therapist is able to use this information to formulate a treatment strategy.

Depending on which treatment strategy is adopted, the practitioner will proceed to use her thumbs or fingertips if she needs to apply very specfic pressure to a pressure point. If a more generalized area requires working on, she is more likely to use her palms. If particularly strong pressure is needed, then the forearms, elbows, knees or feet may be used.

Fig 1 shows the palms being used to feel for energetic blockages.

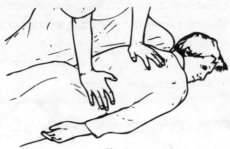

Fig 1

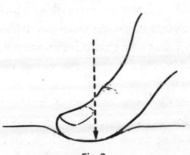

Fig 2

Fig 2 shows the thumb being used to give sustained pressure to a pressure point. Sustained pressure given at right angles to a pressure point has the effect of revitalizing that area (see page 5).

Fig 3 illustrates the use of forearms, elbows, knees and feet.

HOW DOES SHIATSU WORK?

Shiatsu works on the concept that Shiatsu techniques applied to areas of your body will improve overall health. The manner in

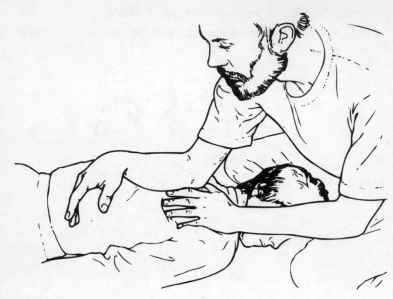

Fig 3a

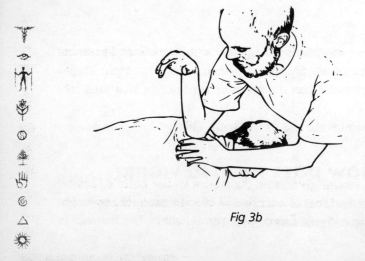

Fig 3b

PRINCIPLES OF SHIATSU

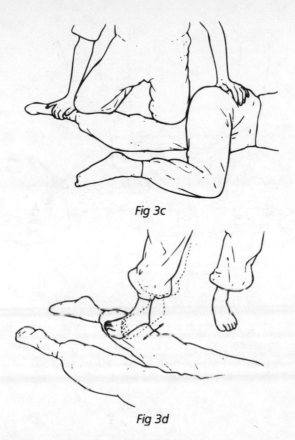

Fig 3c

Fig 3d

which Shiatsu is applied determines its precise effect. There are three broad categories of Shiatsu technique:

Tonification
Dispersal
Calming

Sustained pressure given at right angles to the body's surface will increase the level of energy and blood circulating through that area. This is 'tonification' (Fig 4).

PRINCIPLES OF SHIATSU

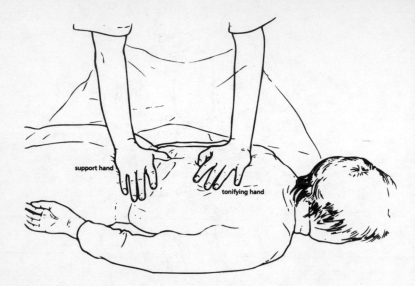

Fig 4: Tonification (perpendicular pressure)

Active techniques such as shaking, rocking, stretching, circling and squeezing disperse blocked or engorged energy and blood. This is called 'dispersal' or 'sedation' (Fig 5).

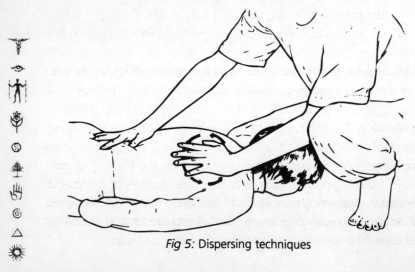

Fig 5: Dispersing techniques

PRINCIPLES OF SHIATSU

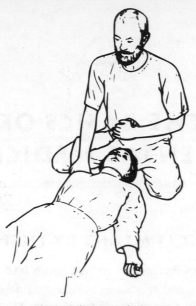

Fig 6: Calming techniques

Light stationary holding with the palm using minimal or no pressure, or very gentle rocking will calm agitated energy. This is called 'calming' (Fig 6).

A Shiatsu session will generally include all three of the above methods, with a bias towards one or other depending upon the type of energetic imbalance predominating.

During all tonification techniques, most calming techniques and many dispersing techniques, the palm of the other hand will be feeling for reactions to those techniques elsewhere in the body.

Notice in Fig 4 that while the thumb of one hand is 'tonifying' the pressure point, the other hand, known as the support hand, is applying palm pressure somewhere else on the body. The purpose of the support hand is to feel for the reaction of the thumb pressure within the body as a whole. This is because tonification of certain pressure points not only affects the area around that point, but has an effect throughout the body and mind.

PRINCIPLES OF SHIATSU

THE BASICS OF
ORIENTAL MEDICINE

WHAT IS MEANT BY ENERGY?

Shiatsu takes its theoretical basis from traditional Oriental philosophy and medicine, which considers everything in nature to be a manifestation of energy. That which is solid and substantial, such as the physical body, is seen simply as a more condensed form of energy than that which is insubstantial, such as thought. This idea is basically the same as the way modern physics views the universe.

This all-encompassing energy is called Ki (sometimes spelt Qi or Ch'i). Ki has as many different manifestations as there are phenomena in nature. For example, desire, bones, and the ability to run are all forms of Ki; just as modern physics sees them all as 'energy'. Blood and Body Fluids are seen as more material forms of Ki, whereas thoughts are considered to be Ki in its most subtle and insubstantial form. Having explained that, I will henceforth reserve the word 'Ki' for that energy which holds things together and in place (i.e. energetically cohesive force – like 'magnetism') and for that power which enables movement. Therefore, the ability to move around is directly related to the quantity and free circulation of Ki within the body. Likewise, the pumping action of the heart and movement of blood is also dependent upon Ki.

Bodily Ki, Mind, Blood and Body Fluids all influence each other, so that an imbalance in one will, at some level, affect the interplay of every other. In areas where Ki is blocked, blood flow and Body Fluids will slow up. Where blood flow is restricted, Ki will be diminished. When morale is low and our chests hollow in despair, the Ki and blood to the chest muscles will be lacking.

In short, three main factors are important to remember when considering Ki within the body:

- Ki quantity and Ki flow determines our ability to function and move

- Ki moves blood, and blood follows Ki

- Ki follows the Mind and reacts to our emotions

Later on we shall see how Shiatsu, by directly working with Ki, can positively influence our energy levels, blood circulation and any emotional imbalances.

CHANNELS AND THE CIRCULATION OF KI

Ki links all functions and organs of the body through a system of interconnecting Channels (sometimes called Meridians). The Channels are the same as those used in acupuncture, although Shiatsu recognizes some additional extensions to their distribution. A Ki Channel flows partly inside the body to connect with the organs, and partly near the surface of the body. It is the Channel sections which are near the surface of the body which are accessible to Shiatsu technique. All the Ki Channels are ultimately connected up to each other to form a continuous circuit of Ki flow, animating all parts of the body as it passes through. The aim of Shiatsu is to keep the Ki flowing without restriction.

Many Channels have been identified, fourteen of which contain pressure points which influence Organs and associated bodily functions. Twelve of the Channels are named after the Organ through which they pass – Kidney Channel, Bladder Channel, Liver Channel and so on.

The body and mind are not mutually exclusive, which means that by affecting the body we are able to affect the mind, and vice versa. According to Oriental Medicine, each Channel has correspondences to aspects of the mind and emotions as well as having physical correspondences within the body. For example, the Channel which runs through the Kidneys influences willpower, drive and the capacity for fear; it is a major factor in the growth and strength of bones, nerves and brain tissue and it also influences the balance of water and minerals within the body.

These Channels are waves or currents of Ki which permeate the body, much like the way water currents resulting from feeder streams or thermal activity permeate a lake. The water currents will persist as long as the feeder streams remain unblocked and contain water.

The following pages illustrate the locations of these Channels. The broken lines indicate the pathway of the Channel, whereas the dotted lines show extensions to the channel, i.e. areas which when pressed or stretched, influence the main Channel.

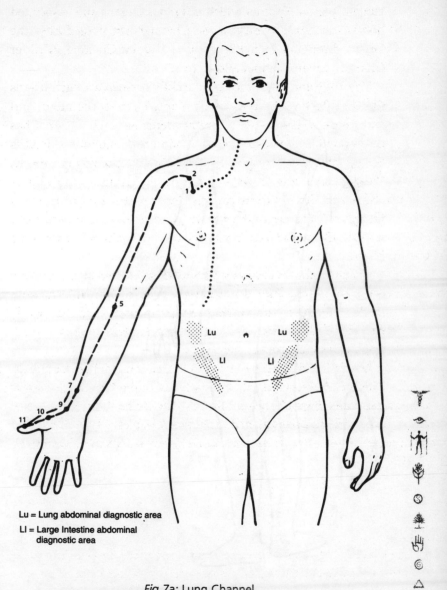

Lu = Lung abdominal diagnostic area
LI = Large Intestine abdominal
     diagnostic area

Fig 7a: Lung Channel

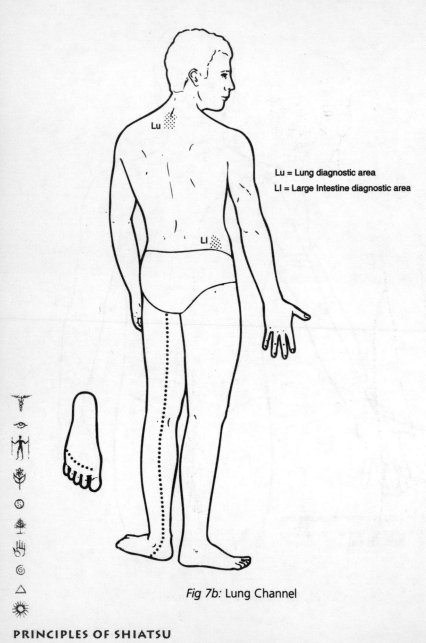

Lu = Lung diagnostic area
LI = Large Intestine diagnostic area

Fig 7b: Lung Channel

PRINCIPLES OF SHIATSU

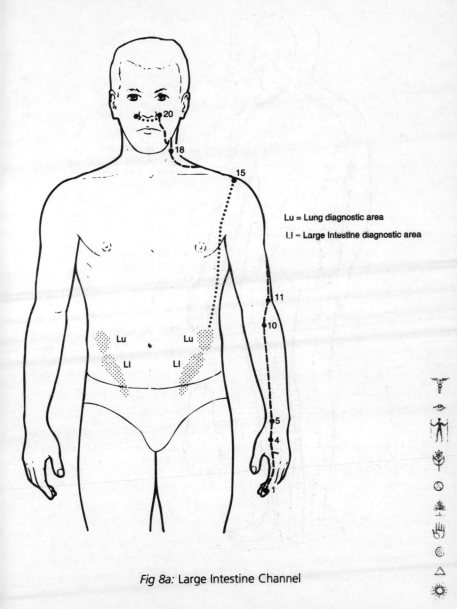

Lu = Lung diagnostic area

LI – Large Intestine diagnostic area

Fig 8a: Large Intestine Channel

PRINCIPLES OF SHIATSU

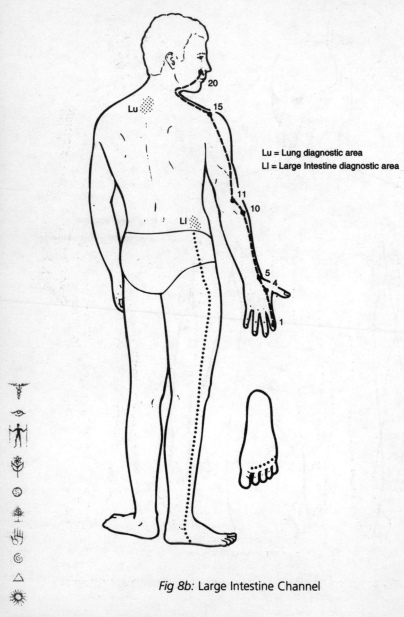

Lu = Lung diagnostic area
LI = Large Intestine diagnostic area

Fig 8b: Large Intestine Channel

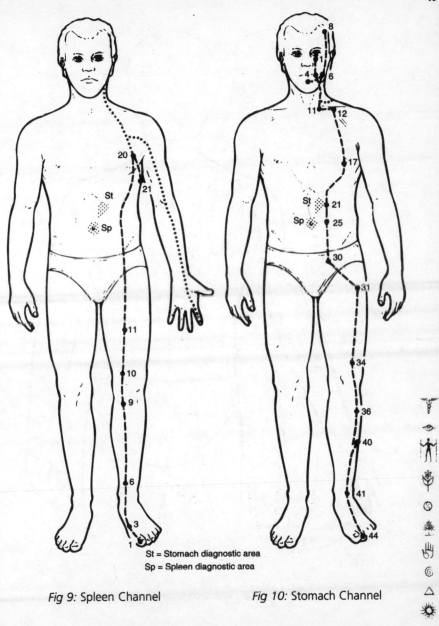

St = Stomach diagnostic area
Sp = Spleen diagnostic area

Fig 9: Spleen Channel

Fig 10: Stomach Channel

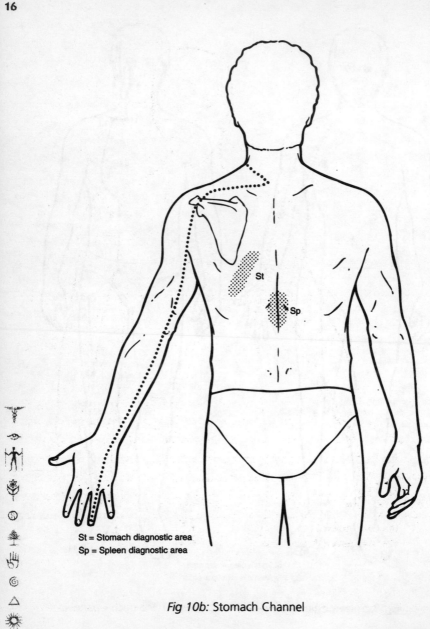

St = Stomach diagnostic area
Sp = Spleen diagnostic area

Fig 10b: Stomach Channel

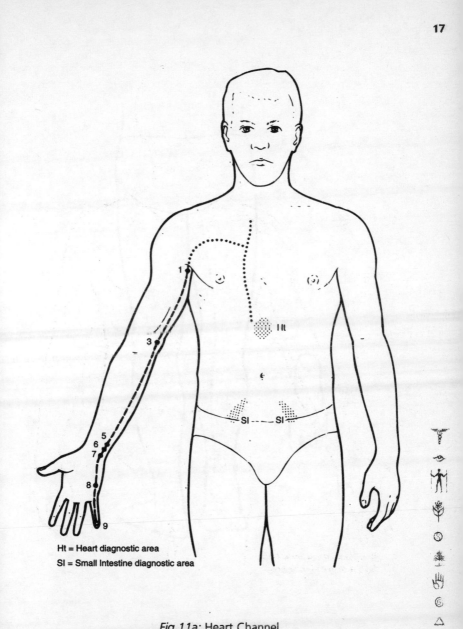

Ht = Heart diagnostic area
SI = Small Intestine diagnostic area

Fig 11a: Heart Channel

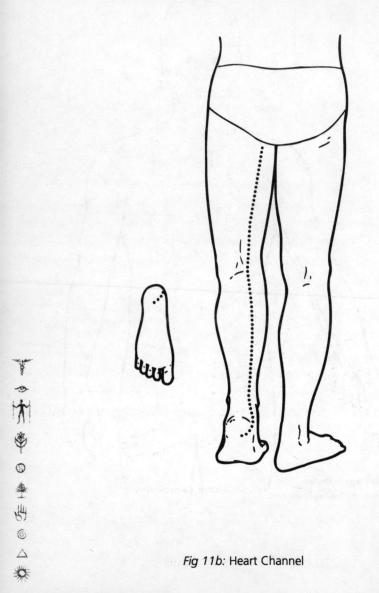

Fig 11b: Heart Channel

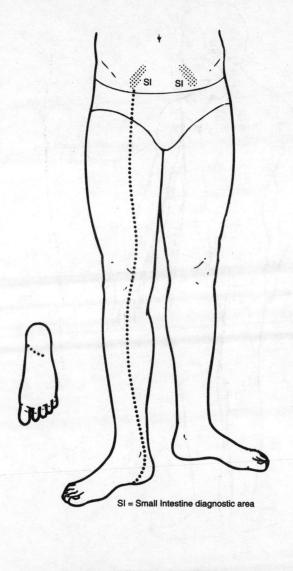

SI = Small Intestine diagnostic area

Fig 12a: Small Intestine Channel

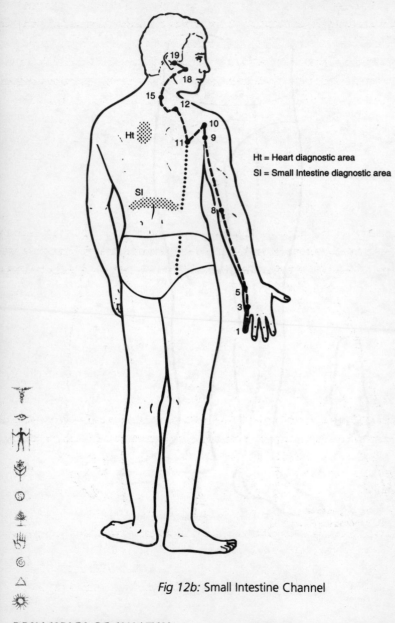

Ht = Heart diagnostic area
SI = Small Intestine diagnostic area

Fig 12b: Small Intestine Channel

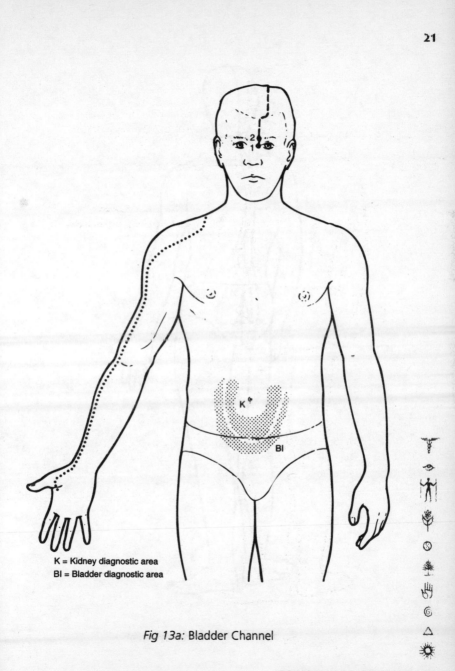

K = Kidney diagnostic area
Bl = Bladder diagnostic area

Fig 13a: Bladder Channel

PRINCIPLES OF SHIATSU

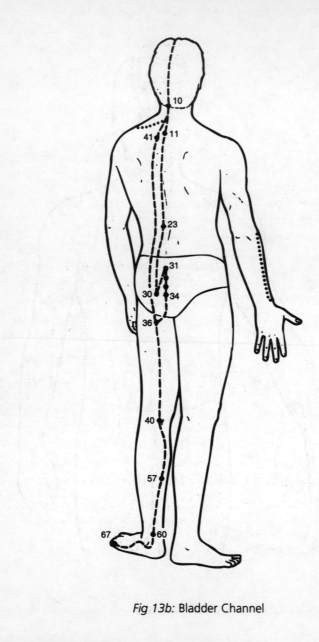

Fig 13b: Bladder Channel

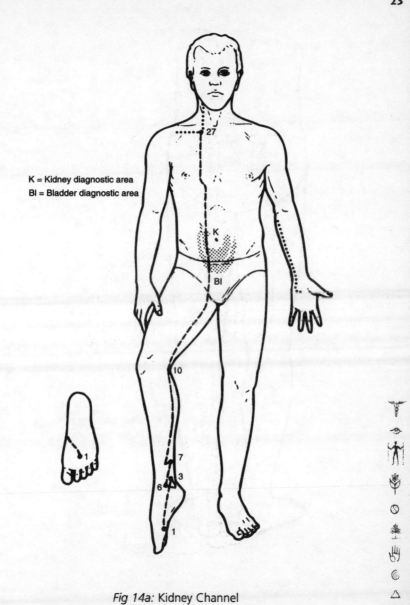

K = Kidney diagnostic area
Bl = Bladder diagnostic area

Fig 14a: Kidney Channel

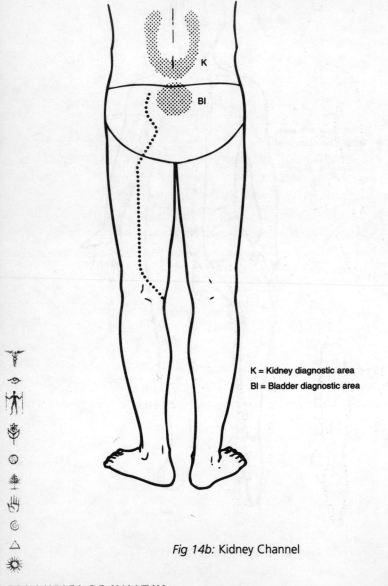

K = Kidney diagnostic area
Bl = Bladder diagnostic area

Fig 14b: Kidney Channel

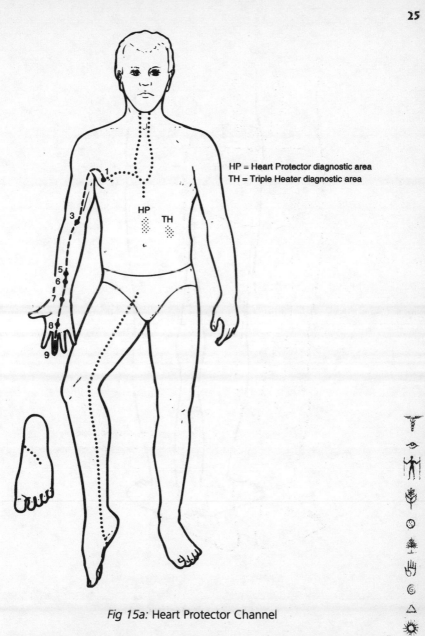

HP = Heart Protector diagnostic area
TH = Triple Heater diagnostic area

Fig 15a: Heart Protector Channel

PRINCIPLES OF SHIATSU

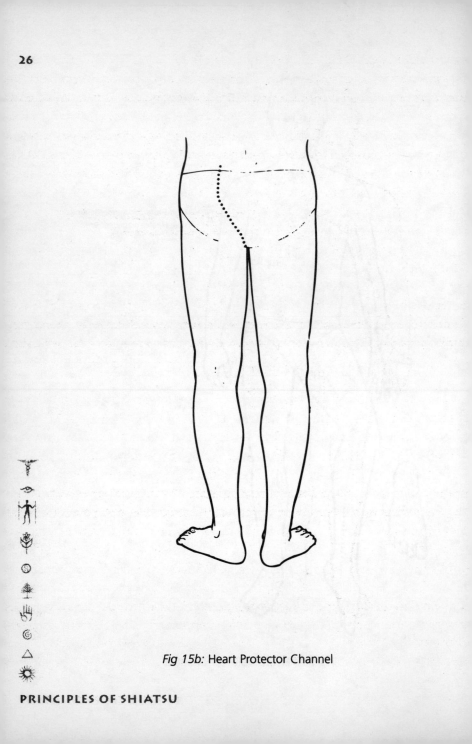

Fig 15b: Heart Protector Channel

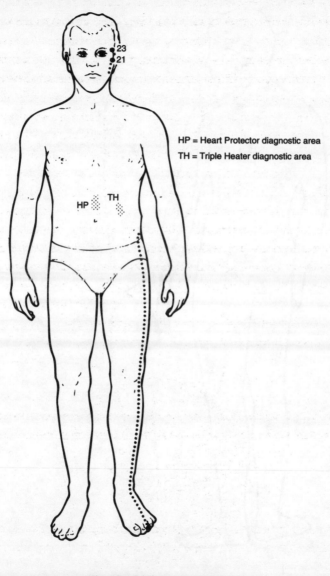

HP = Heart Protector diagnostic area
TH = Triple Heater diagnostic area

Fig 16a: Triple Heater Channel

PRINCIPLES OF SHIATSU

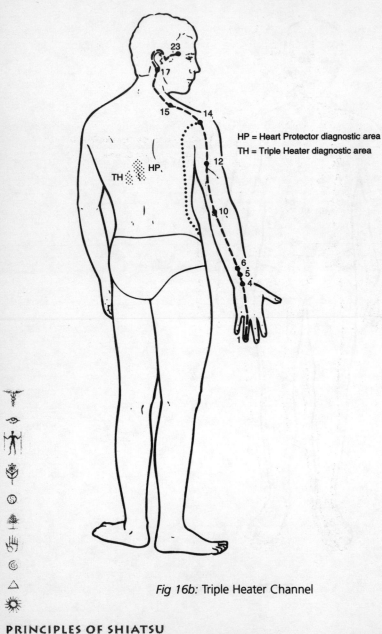

HP = Heart Protector diagnostic area
TH = Triple Heater diagnostic area

Fig 16b: Triple Heater Channel

PRINCIPLES OF SHIATSU

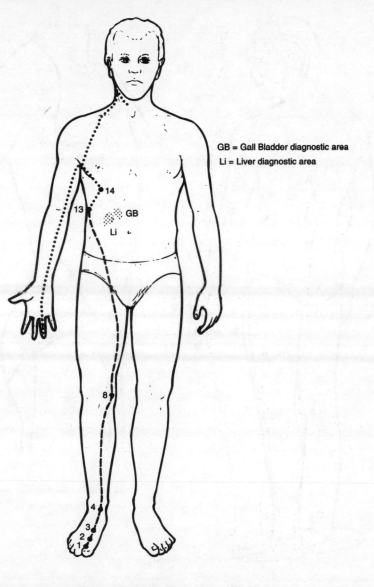

GB = Gall Bladder diagnostic area
Li = Liver diagnostic area

14

13

GB

Li

8

4

3

2

1

Fig 17: Liver Channel

PRINCIPLES OF SHIATSU

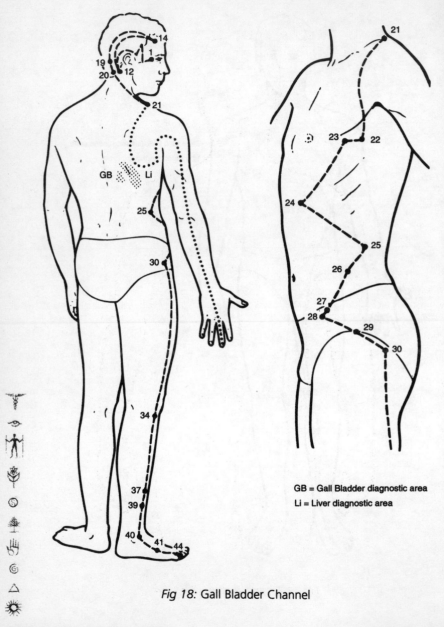

GB = Gall Bladder diagnostic area
Li = Liver diagnostic area

Fig 18: Gall Bladder Channel

PRINCIPLES OF SHIATSU

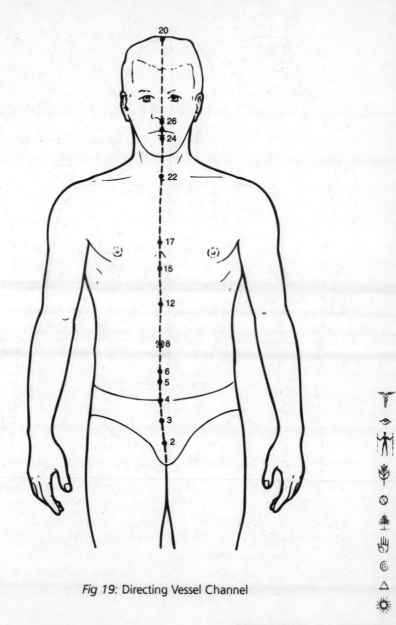

Fig 19: Directing Vessel Channel

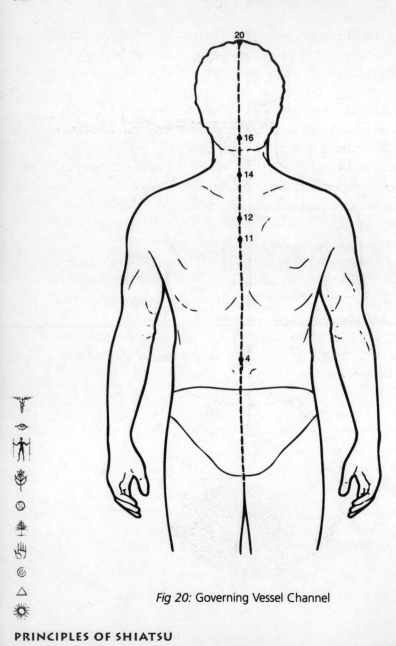

Fig 20: Governing Vessel Channel

YIN/YANG

Keeping the Ki flowing along the Channels requires harmony between all aspects of your personality and your body. The concept of harmony and balance in Oriental Medicine is expressed through the idea of Yin/Yang. Yin/Yang is basically the two sides of everything in the universe. Everything has both a front and a back, neither of which can exist without the other. As such, everything in nature has both Yin and Yang qualities – nothing is totally one or the other. Warm water for example, is more Yang than ice but more Yin compared to steam.

Yin is analogous to the shady side of a slope. It is associated with such qualities as cold, darkness, rest, passivity, responsiveness, downwardness, inwardness, decrease and femininity. Yang, by contrast, can be compared to the sunny side of a slope. It is associated with warmth, brightness, activity, movement, vigour, excitement, stimulation, upwardness, outwardness, increase and masculinity.

Fig 21, the Chinese symbol for Yin/Yang clearly illustrates that Yin and Yang interpenetrate each other and contain the seed of each other.

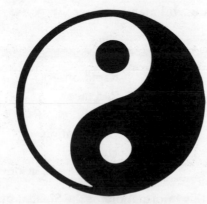

Fig 21: Yin/Yang

Many comparisons of Yin/Yang are listed below:

Yin	Yang
Shade	Brightness
Female	Male
Moon	Sun
Rest	Activity
Material	Immaterial
Contraction	Expansion
Soft	Hard

Within the body, Yin/Yang manifest in the following way:

Yin	Yang
Front	Back
Organ's substance	Energy supplying organs
Interior organs	Exterior tissues – skin, muscles
Blood, body fluids	Ki
Moist	Dry
Slow	Rapid
Cold	Hot
Sinking	Rising

Clinically, Yin/Yang will manifest thus:

Yin	Yang
Chronic disease	Acute disease
Gradual onset	Rapid onset
Pale face	Red face
Not thirsty	Thirsty
Loose stools	Constipation
Cold	Heat
Sleepiness	Restlessness, insomnia

The relevance of this information for the Shiatsu practitioner is that it facilitates diagnosis. We can assess the person as having

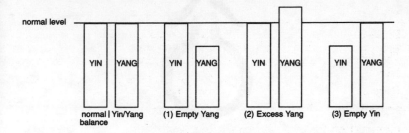

Fig 22: Yin/Yang combinations

insufficient Yang (Empty Yang), too much Yang (Excess Yang), insufficient Yin (Empty Yin), or too much Yin (Excess Yin). Excess Yin is comparatively rare as it can only occur from exposure to extreme cold.

Excess Yang causes the body to generate heat and become overactive. However, heat and dryness can be generated because of a lack of cool, moist Yin energy in the body, allowing the hotter Yang to predominate. This is Empty Yin. Empty Yang results in coldness and lethargy. Fig 22 illustrates these important comparisons.

The Shiatsu therapist can help balance out such discrepancies in Yin/Yang balance by smoothing or strengthening the Ki flow within the Channels, and by stimulating specific pressure points which have documented effects upon the body's Yin/Yang ratio.

TSUBO

At specific locations along a Channel, Ki makes a closer connection to the surface. These are the points where the Ki is traditionally stimulated in acupuncture using needles or in Shiatsu using touch. These points are known as Acupoints or

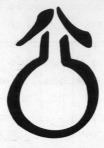

Fig 23: Tsubo

Tsubos and can be likened metaphorically to a vase with a neck narrower than its belly. The Chinese and Japanese character for Tsubo illustrates this concept nicely (Fig 23).

The vase representation is more than metaphoric in that if we could encapsulate the energetic vortex of a Tsubo in the visible spectrum, it would indeed probably look just like the diagram in Fig 24.

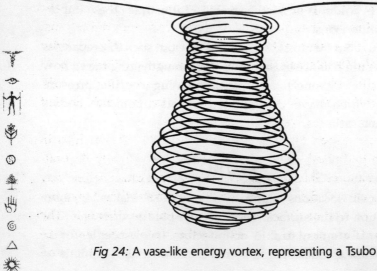

Surface of body

Fig 24: A vase-like energy vortex, representing a Tsubo

PRINCIPLES OF SHIATSU

Unlike acupuncture, Shiatsu makes a direct tactile connection to the Channel's Ki flow, rather than to the classical Tsubos alone. Experience reveals that in addition to the fixed Tsubos, all of which have names, numbers and documented actions on the body and mind when stimulated, there are 'transient Tsubos' which come and go along the Channels between the fixed Tsubos. These transient Tsubos reflect either a lack of Ki at their location, or a build-up of Ki pressure due to a blockage in the Ki flow. Where the Ki is lacking, nearby Tsubos will feel lifeless and empty, lacking vitality and elasticity. Where the Ki is blocked and consequently overcrowded, there will be a feeling of fullness, tightness and constriction; pain is often present. Sometimes the full blocked areas will feel warm whereas the deficient areas will feel cold.

KYO AND JITSU

In Shiatsu terminology, fullness or blockage in a Channel or Tsubo is referred to as 'Jitsu', whereas emptiness is known as 'Kyo'. Kyo and Jitsu thus refer to the energetic quality of the Channel rather than the Yin/Yang balance within the internal Organs. It is easiest to think of Kyo/Jitsu as the body's exterior reaction to its internal Yin/Yang imbalances. Kyo/Jitsu refer to the relative states of emptiness and fullness in the Channels, and therefore do not exist or mean anything in the absence of the other. Like Yin/Yang they are not 'absolutes'.

You can expect any Channel to err towards Kyo or Jitsu in relation to any other. The whole pattern is constantly fluctuating. The aim of Shiatsu is to discover the root cause behind any acute or chronic disharmony and attempt to stabilize it via tonification of Kyo or dispersal of Jitsu within the Channels. The Jitsu areas are easy to find because they feel 'active' and protrude from the surface. Kyo areas are more difficult to find because they exhibit little or no reaction, and are hidden below the surface.

Sensitive Shiatsu done all over the body would highlight these Kyo/Jitsu deviations and re-harmonize the general level and flow of Ki. However, a good professional practitioner would be able to assess which Channel is most lacking in Ki, and which one is most blocked. By balancing these two off against each other, all the other imbalances in all the other Channels will tend to balance themselves out.

The chart in Fig 25 gives a comparison of Kyo/Jitsu.

Kyo	*Jitsu*
Below surface	Protruding from surface
Less obvious	More obvious
Passive resistance or no resistance	Active resistance
Empty – requires filling	Full – requires emptying/ dispersing
Underactive, leading to stiffness or flaccidity	Hyperactive, leading to congestion, blockage and impenetrability
Slower to respond	Immediate response
Underlying cause	Manifests as symptoms
Requires deep, sustained connection	Requires light, superficial connection, or none at all
Its tonification affects the whole person	Its dispersal affects localized body areas

Fig 25: Comparison of Kyo/Jitsu

Most Channels are named after an organ. However, the Oriental Medical view of each organ is wider in connotation than in Western Medicine. Try not to equate these functions with the western concept of organ function. That will only lead to total confusion. The term for Organ as defined by Traditional Oriental Medicine is 'Zangfu'.

The twelve Zangfu Organs are classified in pairs. Each pair contains one Yin (or 'Zang') and one Yang '(or 'Fu') Organ. Thus we have six pairs of Zangfu:

Yin (Zang) Organ	Yang (Fu) Organ
Kidneys	Bladder
Liver	Gall Bladder
Heart	Small Intestines
Heart Protector	Triple Heater
Spleen	Stomach
Lungs	Large Intestines

When referring to organs in Oriental Medicine we will use a capital letter to differentiate them from the western meaning, e.g. Kidneys, Heart etc. The same applies to any other concepts, which may take on a slightly different meaning from that which you are used to in everyday language, e.g. Blood, Body Fluids.

Oriental Medicine describes each Organ and its functions in relation to: a) Ki, Blood, and Body Fluids; b) a specific body tissue; c) a sense organ; d) an emotion; e) a climate. The following few pages describe these relationships.

THE INTERNAL ORGANS IN RELATION TO KI

THE LUNGS GOVERN KI AND RESPIRATION

When air is inhaled, the Lungs extract fresh 'pure' Ki from it. On exhalation, stale Ki is expelled, along with waste gases. This maintains the continual renewal and freshness of bodily Ki.

Ki extracted from food by the Spleen combines with the Ki from air to be circulated through the Channels. It is also circulated under the skin as Defensive Ki (protecting us from weather extremes and pathogenic organisms, and also warming the skin and muscles).

The Large Intestine also has a role in the formation of Defensive Ki.

THE SPLEEN EXTRACTS KI FROM FOOD

When food is ingested, the Spleen extracts Ki from it. This process intimately involves the Stomach, because the Stomach is said to 'rot and ripen' ingested food, meaning that it prepares it for Ki extraction by the Spleen. The Spleen sends some of this Food-Ki to the Lungs to combine with Ki extracted from air, which is then circulated through the Channels, and under the skin as Defensive Ki. The Spleen also sends some Food-Ki to the Heart to enrich the Blood and give it impetus.

THE KIDNEYS STORE KI AS 'ESSENCE', AND CONTROL THE RECEPTION OF KI

Ki is stored by the Kidneys as 'Essence', which is a 'denser', more Yin state of Ki, responsible for growth and reproduction. Most of this Essence is inherited from our parents, but can be supplemented by Ki extracted from food by the Spleen.

The Ki extracted from air by the Lungs is anchored by the Kidneys. If the Kidneys fail to do this, Ki will become trapped in the chest and asthma may develop.

The Liver ensures that Ki flows smoothly through the Channels and to the organs. If it fails to do this, Ki stagnates, obstructing the body functions and causing the mind to become tense and frustrated. On the other hand, tension and frustration can block Ki flow and upset the Liver.

THE INTERNAL ORGANS IN RELATION TO BLOOD

THE HEART GOVERNS BLOOD

This means that if the Heart is strong, it can pump Blood efficiently and in abundance throughout the body. Therefore, it plays the major role in circulation. The Heart is assisted in this function by the Heart Protector. The Lungs also assist the Heart in this function by providing Ki for the maintenance of blood vessels.

THE LIVER STORES BLOOD

The Liver regulates the amount of Blood in circulation according to the levels of physical activity. During rest, a large proportion of Blood flows to the Liver to be stored. During physical activity, the Blood returns to general circulation, ensuring adequate energy, and nourishing of the joints, skin, nails and other body parts.

THE SPLEEN IS THE SOURCE OF BLOOD, AND HOLDS BLOOD

Because the Spleen is the main organ of digestion, it helps transform ingested food and drink into Blood. It 'controls' Blood by keeping it in the blood vessels. Failure of this function can result in haemorrhage or excessive menstrual bleeding.

THE INTERNAL ORGANS IN RELATION TO BODY FLUIDS

THE LUNGS DISPERSE BODY FLUIDS AND REGULATE WATER PASSAGES

The Lungs influence the excretion of sweat and urine. Firstly, they spread Body Fluids all over the body to the skin, moistening it, and regulating the opening and closing of the pores. As such, the Lungs influence sweating. Water retention (oedema) in the face may result if this function is impaired. The Lungs also help the Bladder's function of excreting urine.

THE SPLEEN SEPARATES AND TRANSPORTS FLUIDS

The Spleen separates the usable part of ingested fluids from the unusable part. The usable or 'clean' part goes upwards to the Lungs for distribution to the skin. The unusable or 'dirty' part goes downwards to the Small Intestine for further refinement. If this function of the Spleen is impaired, the fluids may accumulate to create Dampness, too much Phlegm, or cause water retention (oedema).

The Stomach assists the Spleen in the extraction of fluids from food to make Body Fluids.

THE KIDNEYS GOVERN WATER

The Kidneys may be thought of as a 'gate' which opens and closes to control the flow of fluid secretion. When the warming, more energizing function of the Kidneys (Kidney-Yang) is deficient, the gate is too open, leading to copious, clear urination. When the cooling, more nourishing function of the Kidneys (Kidney-Yang) is deficient, the gate is too closed, leading to scanty, dark urination.

The storage and excretion of urine is physically performed by

THE HEART CONTROLS SWEAT

Body Fluids enter the blood vessels to thin down the Blood when it gets too thick. Conversely, Body Fluids leave the Blood if the Blood gets too thin. Thus there is a constant interchange between Blood and Body Fluids. This function is controlled by the Heart. Continuous excessive sweating will therefore lead to a loss of Body Fluids and consequent deficiency of Blood. Weakness in the Heart-Ki may result in spontaneous sweating.

THE INTERNAL ORGANS IN RELATION TO THE TISSUES

THE HEART CONTROLS THE BLOOD VESSELS AND MANIFESTS IN THE COMPLEXION

As part of its function of governing the Blood, the Heart also controls the blood vessels. A healthy Heart will mean strong blood vessels, healthy circulation, and consequently a lustrous, rosy complexion.

THE LIVER CONTROLS THE SINEWS AND MANIFESTS IN THE NAILS

Because the Liver regulates the amount of Blood in circulation, it controls the nourishment of the tendons and ligaments, ensuring smooth movement of joints and ease of muscular action. Failure of this Liver function results in stiffness, or even tremors. The Gall Bladder also relates to the sinews. Whereas the Liver nourishes the sinews with Blood, the Gall Bladder provides them with sufficient Ki to ensure their proper movement. The Liver's regulation of Blood also determines the amount of nourishment reaching the nails. A lack of Blood in circulation therefore results in cracked, dry and indented nails.

THE LUNGS CONTROL THE SKIN AND BODY HAIR

Because the Lungs disperse Ki to the skin and ensure that the body surface receives adequate nourishment and moisture, the Lungs are said to control the skin and body hair. If the Body Fluids are properly dispersed by the Lungs, the skin will be lustrous and the hair shiny. If not, the skin will become dry and body hair brittle and withered.

THE SPLEEN CONTROLS THE MUSCLES AND MANIFESTS IN THE LIPS

The Spleen extracts nourishment from food and transports it to the body parts, including the muscles, ensuring their strength and development.

Food passing the lips is the first stage of digestion. For this reason, the lips are closely connected to the Spleen. Therefore dry, cracked or pale lips show that Spleen-Ki is weak.

THE KIDNEYS CONTROL THE BONES AND MANIFEST IN THE HAIR

The strength and growth of bones depends on the strength of the Essence which enables growth. Because the Kidneys store this Essence (which equates with the genetic structure of the body) they therefore control the bones and teeth. The bone marrow, in Oriental Medicine, includes the brain, spinal cord, and nerves. Thus, the Kidneys control these also.

The hair on the head also depends upon the Essence and therefore the Kidneys for normal growth. Weak Essence reflects in thin, brittle and greying hair.

THE INTERNAL ORGANS AND
THE SENSE ORGANS

THE HEART CONTROLS THE TONGUE AND TASTE

Although the tongue shows the condition of all the Organs, it has particular bearing on that of the Heart. The Heart therefore controls the sense of taste and affects speech.

THE LIVER CONTROLS THE EYES AND SIGHT

The Liver nourishes and maintains the eyes because it regulates the amount of Blood in circulation and because a deep pathway of the Liver Channel enters the eyes. If this Liver function is impaired, there may be dry, gritty eyes, poor vision and the presence of spots or 'floaters'. However, many other organs also influence the eyes, so that not all eye problems are caused by the Liver.

THE LUNGS CONTROL THE NOSE AND SMELL

The Lungs are intimately connected with the breath. The nose is the gateway of the breath. Therefore the Lungs control the nose and the sense of smell. However, smell is also influenced by the Spleen. The nose becomes blocked when the Ki of the Lungs is weak.

THE SPLEEN CONTROLS THE MOUTH AND TASTE

The Spleen influences the sense of taste as well as a feeling of appetite. It relates to the mouth because chewing is the first stage in the transformation of food. Food transformation is a function of the Spleen, assisted by the Stomach.

THE KIDNEYS CONTROL THE EARS AND HEARING

The Essence which is stored in the Kidneys to enable growth and reproduction is also required to enable the ears to function. Therefore the ears and hearing relate most closely to the Kidneys.

THE INTERNAL ORGANS AND MENTAL FACULTIES

THE HEART HOUSES THE MIND

The Heart influences the Mind, in that it governs mental activity, emotions, consciousness, memory, thinking and sleep. This is because the Heart controls the Blood. When Blood is abundant and freely circulating to all the Organs and the brain, the mental faculties are clear. This function of influencing the Mind is shared with the Heart Protector. However, although the Heart and Heart Protector govern the broad spectrum of Mind functions, the other Organs influence aspects of these functions, as described below.

THE LIVER HOUSES THE ETHEREAL SOUL

The ethereal soul is the part of one's being considered to survive after death to return to the world of immaterial existence. During life it provides us with our capacity for vision and planning. The emotion related to the Liver is anger.

The Liver is paired with the Gall Bladder, which controls judgement and the capacity to make decisions. Decision making is also influenced by the Small Intestine. Whereas the Gall Bladder gives us the courage and initiative to make decisions, it is the Small Intestine which provides the clarity of mind to make decisions.

THE LUNGS HOUSE THE CORPOREAL SOUL

The corporeal soul is that which enables us to feel sensations. Consequently it is the most physical and material aspect of our 'soul'. Since it deals with sensations felt in the present, it enables us to experience 'reality' which is the sum total of experiences perceived and felt 'now' rather than those remembered or anticipated. The emotion related to the Lungs is sadness or grief.

The willpower which is under the influence of the Kidneys provides the instinct for survival, determination and the drive to procreate. The emotion related to the Kidneys is fear.

The Gall Bladder also has an influence on willpower and drive insofar as it gives the courage and initiative to turn the Kidneys' drive into decisive action.

THE SPLEEN HOUSES THOUGHT

The Spleen influences the process of thinking, analysing, concentrating and studying, ensuring strong powers of reasoning and memory. A weakness in the Spleen-Ki will result in unclear thought processes and overthinking. The emotion related to the Spleen is pensiveness and worry.

NOTE:

The Triple Heater, unlike the other Zangfu Organs, is an 'Organ' which relates to no particular anatomical structure. It is easiest to consider it a catalyst for the functions of all the other Organs.

The following format explains the Organs and their functions together.

THE KIDNEYS

The Kidneys store Ki as 'Essence' which governs birth, growth and reproduction. In particular, the Essence controls bones, teeth, the brain, the spinal cord and nerves. (This is expressed as 'producing Marrow' in Oriental Medicine). The Essence also enables the ears to function, and the hair to remain healthy and abundant.

Because the Kidney Essence is necessary for reproduction, the Kidneys give us the 'drive' to procreate, plus the willpower and instinct for survival.

The Kidneys provide the Ki to transform fluids unto urine,

and to control the flow of urine. As such they are said to govern water. They also influence defecation because they control the opening and closing of the anus as well as the urethra (i.e. the two lower orifices).

Another effect the Kidneys have upon Ki is to 'anchor' the Ki extracted from the air, sent down to them from the Lungs (expressed as 'controlling the reception of Ki').

THE BLADDER

The Bladder is intimately involved with the Kidneys in transforming fluids into urine. It then stores urine and in due course excretes it from the body.

As you can see, the Bladder as a Zangfu Organ has a relatively simple function. However, the Bladder Channel runs

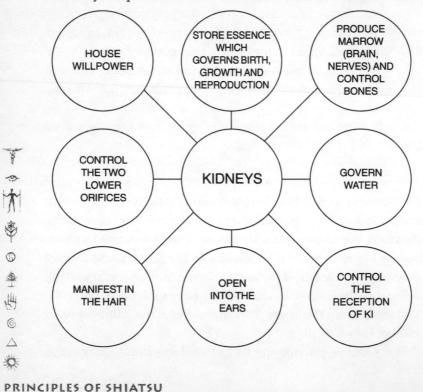

parallel to the vertebral column, in very close proximity to the roots of both the peripheral nerves and the autonomic nervous system, thereby having a strong influence upon them.

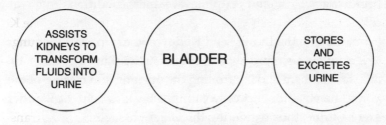

THE LUNGS

The Lungs extract Ki from air, which combines with Ki from food. They subsequently send this Ki through the Channels (and help the Heart to send Ki through the blood

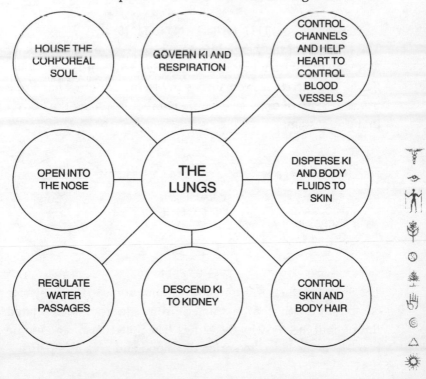

vessels) to energize all the physiological processes of the body. The Lungs also disperse Ki under the skin to provide the body's outer defensive layer, which protects us from pathogenic organisms, and extreme weather conditions such as cold.

In addition, the Lungs send Ki downwards to the Kidneys.

The Lungs also spread Body Fluids to the skin and body hair, moistening them and controlling the opening and closing of the pores, thereby influencing sweating. They also help the Bladder excrete urine, thus regulating the water passages.

Because the nose is the gateway of the breath, the nose, and therefore smell, is controlled by the Lungs.

The Lungs house the corporeal soul, which enables us to feel sensations and 'reality' by allowing us to experience 'now'.

THE LARGE INTESTINE

The function of the Large Intestine is to receive the residue of food and drink from the Small Intestines, re-absorb some of the fluids, and excrete the remains as stools. In addition it has a role in the activity of defensive Ki, therefore influencing the body's immune system.

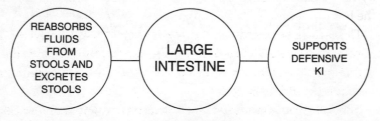

REABSORBS FLUIDS FROM STOOLS AND EXCRETES STOOLS — LARGE INTESTINE — SUPPORTS DEFENSIVE KI

THE SPLEEN

The Spleen extracts Ki from food, sending some to the Lungs for combining with that extracted from air, to be circulated throughout the body by the Lungs. The Spleen also sends some Food-Ki to the Heart to enrich the Blood and give it impetus.

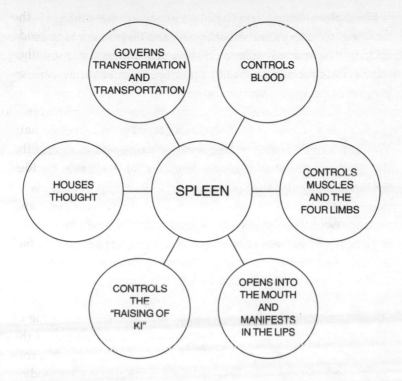

The Blood itself is transformed from ingested food and drink by the Spleen. The Spleen also 'controls' Blood by keeping it in the blood vessels.

The Spleen also separates the 'clean' part of ingested fluids from the 'dirty' part. The 'clean' part goes to the Lungs for distribution to the skin. The 'dirty' part goes to the Small Intestines for further refinement.

The Spleen ensures the strength and development of muscles by extracting nourishment from food and transporting it to the muscles and all other body parts; especially the limbs. It is because food passes the lips in the first stage of digestion that the lips are closely related to the Spleen, as is the mouth and therefore taste.

The Spleen is also responsible for preventing prolapses by 'holding up' organs and other body parts (expressed as 'raising Ki'). In the mental sphere, the Spleen influences thinking, analysing, concentrating and studying, thus ensuring strong powers of reasoning and memory.

THE STOMACH

Through a process akin to fermentation ('rotting and ripening') the Stomach prepares ingested food for Ki extraction by the Spleen. It also helps the Spleen extract fluids from food to make Body Fluids.

Along with the Spleen, the Stomach also controls the transportation of food essences to the entire body, particularly the muscles and limbs.

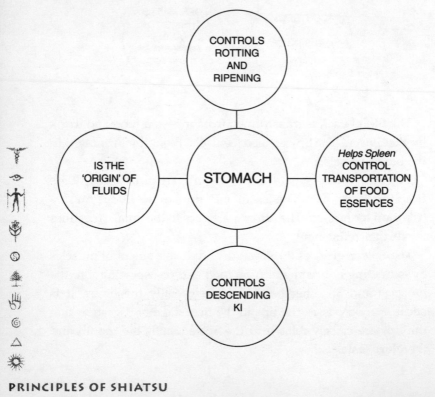

It is the Ki of the Stomach which ensures that food is sent down to the Small Intestines, rather than 'rebelling' upwards to cause belching, hiccups and vomiting (expressed as 'controls descending Ki').

THE HEART

The Heart governs the Blood by giving it impetus to circulate around the body. As part of this function it ensures the health and strength of the blood vessels. Furthermore, by controlling sweating, it regulates the viscosity of Blood through adjusting the amount of Body Fluids within it. A healthy Heart giving good circulation ultimately means a lustrous complexion.

The tongue, which commands a very rich supply of blood, is

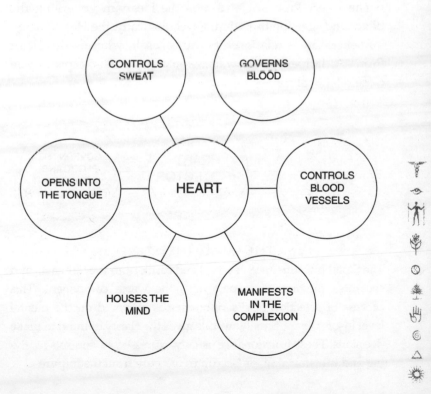

controlled mainly by the Heart. The Heart therefore controls the sense of taste and affects speech.

Finally, is the Heart which has the most general influences on the Mind, governing mental activity, emotions, consciousness, thinking and sleep. Most of the other Organs influence specific nuances of the Mind, but it is the Heart and Blood which 'anchor' the Mind.

THE HEART PROTECTOR

The Heart Protector is closely related to the Heart. It relates to the pericardium, which is the outer covering of the heart organ. It acts like a bodyguard, protecting the Heart from invasion by pathogens, temperature changes and emotional trauma.

The Heart Protector also aids the Heart in governing the Blood and housing the Mind. Psychologically, the Heart energy influences one's relationship with oneself, whereas the Heart Protector influences the way we relate to others, especially in close relationships.

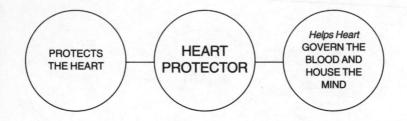

THE SMALL INTESTINE

The Small Intestine receives food and drink from the Stomach, and separates the nutritious part from the waste component. This process of selection or discrimination is mirrored on the mental level insofar as the Small Intestine gives the clarity of mind to make decisions. These functions are usually expressed as 'controls receiving and transforming' or 'separates the pure from the impure'.

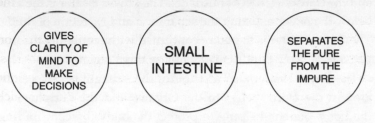

GIVES CLARITY OF MIND TO MAKE DECISIONS

SMALL INTESTINE

SEPARATES THE PURE FROM THE IMPURE

THE TRIPLE HEATER

The Triple Heater is the only 'Organ' which does not equate with a physical organ. Its function is that of a catalyst regulating the functions of Organs in three distinct areas of the body. The thorax is known as the Upper Heater, which gives impetus to the Lung's function of distributing Body Fluids. The Middle Heater is between the diaphragm and the navel, facilitating digestion

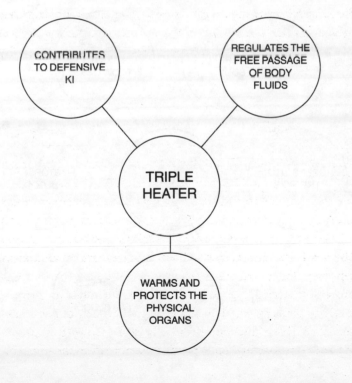

CONTRIBUTES TO DEFENSIVE KI

REGULATES THE FREE PASSAGE OF BODY FLUIDS

TRIPLE HEATER

WARMS AND PROTECTS THE PHYSICAL ORGANS

PRINCIPLES OF SHIATSU

and the transportation of nutrients. The Lower Heater is the area below the navel, assisting the separation and excretion of fluids. The Triple Heater is therefore concerned with regulating the free passage of Body Fluids between these three regions.

The Triple Heater also distributes the strength or 'Ki' generated in the Hara (belly) to the Organs, and the periphery of the body, thereby helping to protect the body (by contributing to the Defensive Ki). It also helps to warm and protect the physical organs.

THE LIVER

The Liver ensures that Ki flows smoothly through the body. In addition it stores much of the Blood during rest, and releases it

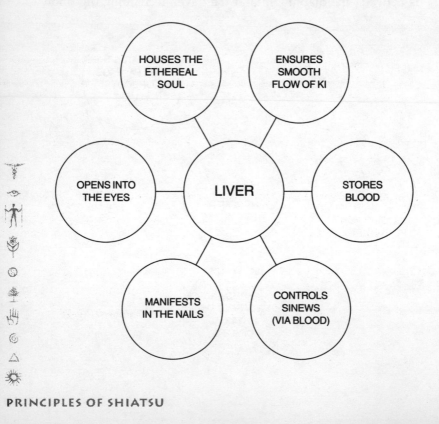

during physical activity, ensuring the nourishment of the body, especially the joints, sinews, eyes and nails.

In the mental sphere, the Liver is said to house the Ethereal Soul, which is our capacity for vision and planning. Unclear vision leads to bad planning, and can result in anger, the emotion associated with the Liver.

THE GALL BLADDER

The Gall Bladder is very closely related to the Liver in function, in that it helps the Liver smooth the flow of Ki. Also, whilst the Liver is nourishing the joints, tendons and ligaments with Blood, the Gall Bladder supplies them with Ki. As a physical structure, the Gall Bladder stores and excretes bile.

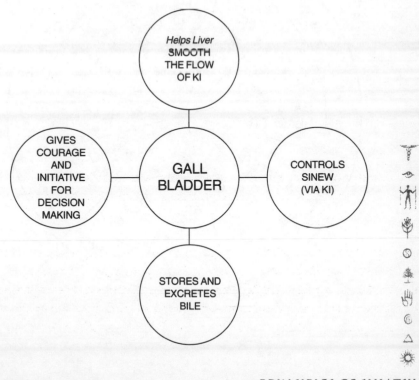

Psychologically, the Gall Bladder complements the Liver's 'plans' by giving the courage and initiative to make decisions. All plans are based upon multiple decisions.

Each Zangfu Organ reaches a peak of activity each day which lasts for a period of two hours. Moreover, each Organ peaks at a different two hour period from any other Organ. Fig 38 illustrates this.

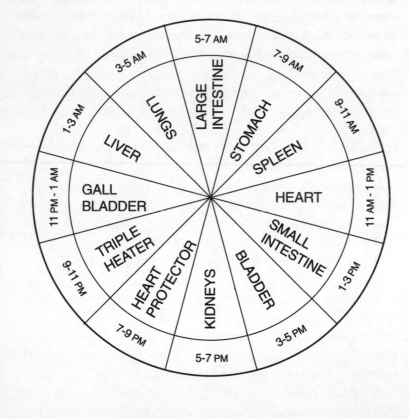

Fig 38: The Chinese Organ Clock

Each pair of Organs and their Channels can be related to one of the Five Elements. The idea of the Five Elements represents a way of comparing human physical and psychological functions with the rhythms of nature. Consequently, we can see the effects of the seasons, colour, tastes and so on upon ourselves and other human beings.

The Five Element model came into being because, to the ancient Chinese, humankind was seen as a reflection, or a microcosm, of the world around us. Most other cultures who live close to the earth also recognize their dependence upon nature, and see their reflection within it. In contrast, modern western civilization has developed a philosophy which is exploitative of the world and its resources. Fortunately, this attitude is slowly beginning to change. The following description will hopefully make the Five Element concept clear to you.

The ancient Chinese viewed life and the universe as an interplay between Yin and Yang, the complementary yet opposite polarities of all phenomena. However, the characteristics of each phenomenon within both ourselves and nature can be described according to five basic qualities or 'Elements', namely: Water, Wood, Fire, Earth and Metal.

Water is the source of life. It has the capacity to flow and yield, and as such can never be eroded like that which is fixed and unyielding. It represents energy in a latent state, as in Winter, when life is waiting and regenerating, to give impetus to the growth of the coming Spring. In us, this impetus manifests as willpower and drive. The Organs and Channels which relate to Water are the Kidneys and Bladder.

Wood is so called because Wood represents trees and indeed all that grows upwards and outwards (both literally and metaphorically) as in Springtime. It represents the energy to grow from a seed and gives the ability to look ahead and plan new possibilities. The associated Organs and Channels are the Liver and Gall Bladder.

Fire is the element of heat and Summer. It is where the expanding energy of Springtime (Wood) has reached its peak. In us it gives enthusiasm, self-awareness and warmth in human relationships. Fire is associated with the Heart, Small Intestines, Heart Protector and Triple Heater.

Earth is analogous to harvest-time with its fertility and mother-like quality of providing abundant nourishment. It relates to the Stomach and Spleen.

Metal includes the Western idea of the Air Element, but it also includes the time when nature replenishes the earth, as in Autumn, when leaves and redundant plant material fall back to the ground to decompose. Metal therefore represents our ability to let go of that which is of no use or can no longer be sustained. The related Organs and Channels are the Lungs and Larger Intestines.

THE CREATION CYCLE

Each Element is said to be the creator or 'mother' of the next insofar as Water nourishes Wood; Wood burns to make Fire; the ashes of Fire decompose into Earth; Earth contains the ores of Metal; and Metal melts into 'Water' (the liquid state).

Each Element generates another and is generated by one. For example, Wood is generated by Water, but generates Fire. This is often expressed as 'Wood is the child of Water and the Mother of Fire'.

THE CONTROL CYCLE

A second cycle exists between alternate Elements exerting a controlling influence. This may be expressed through the image of nature as follows: Wood is cut by Metal; Metal is melted by Fire; Fire is extinguished by Water; Water is channelled by Earth; and Earth is penetrated by Wood.

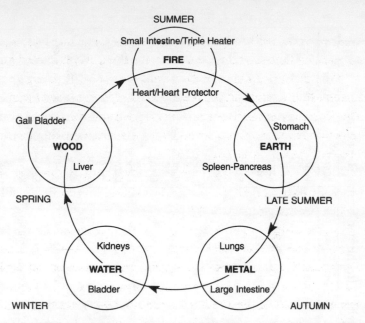

Each Element relates to various phenomena in Nature. The main correspondences are:

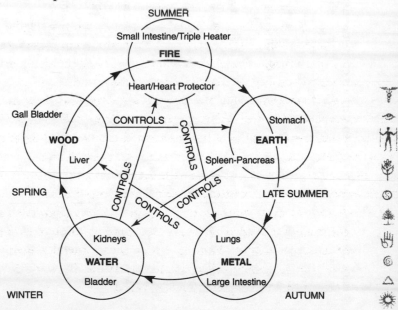

Each Element also relates to various correspondences within the human being. These are:

	Wood	Fire	Earth	Metal	Water
Yin organ & its channel	Liver	Heart/Heart Protector	Spleen	Lung	Kidney
Yang organ & its channel	Gall Bladder	Small Intestine/Triple Heater	Stomach	Large Intestine	Bladder
Tissues	Sinews (Ligaments/Tendons)	Blood vessels	Muscles	Skin	Bones
Sense organs	Eyes	Tongue	Mouth	Nose	Ears
Taste	Sour	Bitter	Sweet	Pungent	Salty
Smell	Rancid	Burned	Sweet/Fragrant	Rank/Rotten	Putrid
Time of day	Morning	Noon	Late afternoon	Evening	Night
Activity	Initiating activity	Peak activity	Decreasing activity	Balance between activity & rest	Rest
Mental capacity	Planning, asserting & controlling	Sensitivity & love	Concentrating & analysing	Taking in & letting go	Willpower & endurance
Emotions	Anger	Joy	Pensiveness, Worry & sympathy	Sadness & grief	Fear
Voice	Shouting/clipped	Laughing	Singing	Weeping	Groaning

PRINCIPLES OF SHIATSU

	Wood	Fire	Earth	Metal	Water
Season	Spring	Summer	Late Summer & short period between each season	Autumn	Winter
Colour	Green	Red	Yellow	White	Black/Blue
Climate	Wind	Heat	Dampness	Dryness	Cold
Stage of Development	Birth	Growth	Transformation	Harvest	Storage

A SUMMARY OF THE ELEMENTS

This summary is designed to put the chart of correspondences into context.

THE WATER ELEMENT

This is associated with night-time and with rest. It provides us with the instinct for survival and the emotion of Fear, as well as the urge to procreate. It is the source of Will in the bodymind and provides it with endurance. Water relates to the Yin Organ of the Kidneys, which house the Essence, the basis of our constitutional strength. Its coupled Yang Organ, also belonging to Water, is the Bladder. A person with a predominance of the Water Element will have a blue tinge to the colour of their face, a groaning sound in their voice, and a slight putrid odour (discernible near the chest or back). They might be slightly timid in character, or inwardly insecure.

THE WOOD ELEMENT

Wood is associated with the morning and with initiating action. It provides the ability to plan, control and assert, and affords the capacity for Anger. Wood relates to the Yin Organ of the Liver, which houses the Ethereal Soul. The Ethereal Soul oversees our individual evolution, and is the source of hope and vision. The Yang Organ which belongs to the Wood Element is the Gall Bladder, the seat of initiative. A person with a predominance of Wood energy will have a shouting quality to the sound of their voice, and a faint rancid odour. They tend to be authoritative, well-organized and frequently irritable.

THE FIRE ELEMENT

This element is associated with noon and activity at its peak. It represents our self-identity and urge to celebrate, bestowing the capacity for Joy and Love. Fire relates to the Yin organ of the Heart, which houses the Mind (Shen). The Mind is the foundation of consciousness and the origin of thought and emotion. It is the most rarified Ki of all. The Fire Element also encompasses the Organs of the Small Intestine, the Heart Protector and the Triple Heater. A person with a predominance of Fire energy will have a red tinge to the colour of their face, a laughing or tremulous quality to the sound of their voice, and a faint scorched odour. They are usually sensitive, excitable or emotionally changeable in nature.

THE EARTH ELEMENT

Earth is associated with the late afternoon and with a decrease in activity. It produces the ability to concentrate and analyse, granting the capacity for Pensiveness. Earth relates to the Yin Organ of the Spleen, which houses Thought. Thought provides the Mind with a logical process, just as the Spleen subjects food to a digestive process. Its coupled Yang Organ is the Stomach, the seat of our ability to listen and absorb. A person with a predominance of Earth energy will have a yellow tinge to the colour of their face, a singing quality to the sound of their voice, and a faintly sweet, or fragrant odour. They are often sympathetic listeners and have a tendency to worry.

This is associated with the evening and a balance between activity and rest. It provides us with a sense of boundary across which we can take in and let go. Connected to the process of 'letting go' is the emotion of the Metal Element: which houses the Corporeal Soul. The Corporeal Soul gives us our 'animal' vitality and inherent optimism; when it is stricken we become despondent. The associated Yang Organ of the Metal Element is the Large Intestine. A person with a predominance of Metal energy will have a white tinge to the colour of their face, a subtle weeping quality to the sound of their voice and a faint rotten odour. Although they can easily feel 'invaded', they quickly become melancholic if they 'lose touch' with those important to them.

THE FIVE ELEMENTS IN SHIATSU

The Five Elements provide a flexible and revealing model for understanding the recipient psychologically, and can lead the attentive Practitioner to an insight into the internal causes of disease.

Each of the emotions within the Five Elements – Fear (Water), Anger (Wood), Joy (Fire), Pensiveness (Earth) and Grief (Metal) – are necessary to complete our character. However, when we get stuck in one or two of these attitudes, they can intensify into passions which dominate the psyche. For example, we can see from our observations of the control cycle that the Water Element 'controls' Fire. If the Water Element becomes afflicted through overwork, the Kidneys (Water) will fail to dampen or 'control' the Heart (Fire). This allows the mind to become overexcited and nervous. Consequently a vague sense of fear from a weakened Water Element coupled with nervousness from an uncontrolled Fire Element will result in anxiety.

Understanding the cause of anxiety from this perspective allows the Shiatsu Practitioner to formulate an appropriate treatment strategy. In this case good results would be achieved from tonifying the Kidneys, as well as dispersing the Heart Channel.

THE CAUSES OF DISEASE

Disease arises when there is an imbalance of Yin/Yang which upsets the normal, smooth and harmonious flow of Ki.

Shiatsu, along with acupuncture and other systems of healing based upon Oriental Medicine, considers the causes of disease to arise either from:

a) Internal causes (i.e. the emotions)
b) External causes (i.e. climatic)
c) Other causes

INTERNAL CAUSES OF DISEASE

Each internal Organ, and therefore its associated Ki Channel, is closely associated with a range of emotions. For example, a disharmony of the Liver may lead to excessive anger, or conversely always feeling angry will tend to block the Liver Channel. Consequently, equal importance is given to the mind and the body when it comes to making a diagnosis.

There are seven basic emotions which make up the Internal Causes of Disease:

- Fear
- Anger
- Overexcitement
- Shock or fright

- Worry
- Pensiveness
- Sadness

In normal circumstances these emotions play a positive role in life. It is only when they become too intense and dominate the psyche that they undermine health.

FEAR

Excessive or prolonged Fear weakens the Kidneys and to some extent disturbs the Heart, leading to anxiety and insecurity. It follows therefore that Shiatsu technique aimed at strengthening the Kidneys will help offset the effects of fear and anxiety and perhaps help provide the energy required for greater self-assurance.

ANGER

Excessive and inappropriate anger adversely affects the Liver. This can result in headaches, diarrhoea, plus stiffness and pain in the joints. Anger, frustration, irritability and resentment prevent Ki from flowing smoothly in the Channels. Shiatsu technique aimed at harmonizing the Liver results in the smoothing of Ki flow in the body, offsetting the effects of anger.

OVEREXCITEMENT

Overexcitement from an abnormal degree of mental stimulation can interfere with the Heart, resulting in emotional instability, anxiety or obsessiveness. Shiatsu to harmonize the Heart will calm the mind very efficiently.

SHOCK

Mental shock scatters the Ki and adversely affects both the Kidneys and the Heart plus, to some extent, the Small

Intestines. The Ki of the Heart is rapidly weakened and requires an input of Kidney energy to support it. This in turn puts a strain on the Kidneys, which require deep tonifying Shiatsu to support them.

WORRY AND PENSIVENESS

Worry and pensiveness (excessive thinking) disrupt the functions of the Spleen and Pancreas and, to some extent, the Lungs. Stress to the Spleen or Pancreas consequently disrupt digestion, whereas the Lungs react to worry by creating difficulties in breathing. The pressures of modern living make worry a common problem. There are many Shiatsu techniques which greatly benefit the breathing, strengthen digestion and harmonize the Spleen and Lungs.

SADNESS

Sadness and grief upset the Lungs even more than worry. If the Lungs are drastically weakened, it will undermine our immune system, of which the Lungs play a major role. Patient tonification of the Lung energy is required and can be very effective indeed.

EXTERNAL CAUSES OF DISEASE

Whereas the Internal Causes of Disease are relatively subtle and arise from within, the External Causes of Disease refer to climatic factors such as Wind, Cold, Heat, Dampness, or Dryness which affect us when our resistance is low, or if we are exposed to extreme weather conditions over a prolonged period. Symptoms caused by Wind predominantly affect the head and may come on suddenly and change rapidly (like gusts of wind). Common symptoms are stiff neck, runny nose, sneezing, coughing and aversion to cold. Wind particularly affects

the Liver Channel, causing stiff and painful joints, wandering
pains and migraines. Shiatsu aimed at dispersing and moving
Ki via the Liver Channel is useful in these circumstances.

Damp entering the body from working and living in damp
conditions weakens the Spleen and Pancreas, thereby upsetting
the digestive process and resulting in an accumulation of fluid
and mucus in the body. Shaitsu aimed at harmonizing the
Spleen is helpful here.

Problems resulting from Cold, Heat or Dryness can be helped
by Shiatsu, but are usually more responsive to acupuncture
when combined with herbal medicine.

OTHER CAUSES OF DISEASE

The Causes of Disease which do not fit into the categories above
are:

- Poor constitution
- Poor dietary habits
- Over-exertion
- Excessive sexual activity
- Trauma
- Parasites and poisons

POOR CONSTITUTION

Your constitution is inherited from your parents and is therefore
largely predetermined. Those with a strong constitution are
able to sustain freedom from ill-health better than those with a
poor constitution. Your constitutional strength determines how
much Ki you have in reserve to combat any stress factors which
might undermine your health.

Factors which diminish your constitutional strength are overwork, excessive sexual activity and drug abuse. If your Shiatsu

therapist feels your symptoms reflect a weakness in constitutional strength, he or she will recommend certain practices which preserve and enhance it. Tai Ji Quan, Yoga and various Taoist forms of meditation all help on this level. However, it is far easier to lose this strength than it is to regain it. The mere act of existing gradually depletes you: that is why you eventually die; because your constitutional Ki reserves run out.

The Kidneys have the most direct role to play in conditions involving constitutional weakness. For this reason, your practitioner would spend a particularly long time tonifying the Kidney Channel and specific Acupoints (Tsubos) known to help this state of being.

POOR DIETARY HABITS

Diet is a major cause or aggravating factor of ill-health in many cases. Shiatsu can help strengthen the digestive system, but any problems which are a direct result of poor dietary habits such as malnutrition cannot be 'cured' until the diet is improved.

OVER-EXERTION

Excessive mental and physical exertion undermine the constitutional strength as described above. In addition, the Spleen, in Oriental Medicine, is especially weakened because physical overwork puts a strain on the muscles which are governed by the Spleen. Shiatsu can do much to offset localized muscular pain resulting from overwork because of the effect it has on promoting circulation and improving muscle tone.

The Spleen energy is also crucial to the process of thinking, therefore excessive mental overwork also tends to weaken the Spleen.

Shiatsu is excellent for dealing with problems resulting from over-exertion and works especially well with a nourishing dietary programme and the use of appropriate tonifying herbs.

What is considered excessive in regard to sexual activity depends upon your constitutional strength. Frequent loss of semen in men, and childbirth in women, both deplete the Ki reserves. Oriental Medicine recommends that sufficient time elapses between ejaculations or births to restore the 'Essence' which underpins your vitality. The more depleted your constitutional strength is, the greater this period of recuperation should be. As you may have guessed, tonifying Shiatsu for the Kidneys would help.

TRAUMA

Trauma refers to physical accident, such as broken bones and bruising. Hospital casualty departments are better at dealing with these things than Shiatsu practitioners. However, for an old injury, Shiatsu is good for increasing Ki and blood circulation, which is often rather blocked where there is scar tissue.

PARASITES AND POISONS

Parasites in the form of worms and poisons are causes of disease which most frequently affect children. Clearly, they are problems which are not easily treated through Shiatsu.

WHAT TO EXPECT WHEN ATTENDING A TREATMENT

THE SHIATSU HEALTH ASSESSMENT

A Shiatsu session lasts between 40 minutes and an hour. The first session you come for may take slightly longer, because a thorough health assessment is usually given at this stage. A health assessment is aimed at pinpointing the underlying cause of your discomfort. It will highlight the aspects of your body and mind which are most likely to be affected if your general vitality drops due to stress or illness.

There are four main categories by which the therapist can assess your state of health or illness:

- Looking
- Asking
- Listening
- Touching

LOOKING

The Shiatsu therapist can see various colourations in your facial hue, facial lines, blemishes and other visible features which give an indication as to where your imbalances lie. Your general

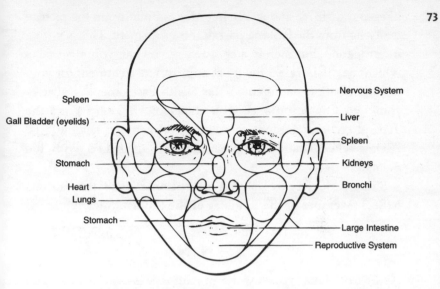

Fig 41: Diagnostic areas of the face

demeanour also adds to this picture. Looking at the tongue can also reveal these imbalances.

This type of information gathering may sound potentially inhibiting, as if the practitioner has the power to read right through you like an open book. However, remember that the practitioner is only assessing your degree of health or disease because that is why you asked for treatment. He or she is not making any judgements about you as a person. You may have come just for relaxation or general invigoration, in which case it is not always necessary to do an extensive health assessment.

ASKING

You may be asked a variety of questions regarding your present symptoms, past symptoms, current and past medication; the health of blood relatives; lifestyle; approximate age; appetite;

likes and dislikes, and so on, in order to build upon the picture evolving from the looking part of the assessment. This is not an interrogation, but merely a chat where you can volunteer facts which may help select the most appropriate treatment for you. All information gathered in the health assessment is strictly confidential in accordance with Shiatsu Society ethics and the general code of conduct common to all genuine healing arts. Always check that your practitioner is registered with the Shiatsu Society.

Shiatsu Society registered practitioners use the initials MRSS (Member of the Register of the Shiatsu Society).

LISTENING

Apart from what you say, the practitioner is also interested in any underlying tones in your voice. As an example, a subtle weeping undertone to your voice might indicate a propensity to dwell upon things which sadden you, which would indicate to the practitioner that your Lungs and Large Intestine Channels might need attention.

As a general rule, a weak quiet voice suggests a general lack of Ki, whereas a loud strong voice indicates strong Ki. Inability to speak, stammering, or curt, clipped replies indicate that the Heart or Liver Channels respectively may need closer attention.

TOUCHING

Since Shiatsu is about touching, it is logical that touch should be the most important aspect of a health assessment.

Experienced practitioners can feel blocked, overactive or insufficient Ki within any area of the body, because it reflects in a certain 'quality' or 'response' to touch. This is particularly clear when working directly upon any of the 14 Channels through which Ki circulates. Where too much Ki causes a blockage along a Channel, the blocked Ki feels like a swelling from which Ki is trying to break out. It feels 'active' and 'hard' in the same way as an over-inflated balloon feels hard; the more you press it, the more it resists. It may not present as an actual swelling, but will definitely feel energetically confined and under pressure. As with a balloon, you would not want to press it too hard for risk of an explosion. An explosion of pain accompanies pressure which is too direct and heavy upon the blocked area. Blocked areas generally like to be left alone. The good practitioner therefore seeks out the areas lacking in Ki, draining Ki from the full areas into the empty areas. This is done by holding steady pressure upon the Tsubos which are most lacking in Ki within the deficient area.

Insufficient Ki in an area makes that area feel empty, lifeless and devoid of zest. It may manifest as a slight flatness to the contours of the body, and may well feel soft, lacking resilience. It may also feel hard, but not the hardness of an inflated balloon or car tyre – this is the hardness of inert matter such as the dried-out crust on top of a stale loaf of bread. Contrast this with a loaf of bread just out of the oven which has the Ki of freshness and warmth to give it some bounce.

Ki may also be insufficient, but trying desperately to fulfil the role of a greater quantity of Ki; rather like two waiters trying desperately to do the job of 12 waiters. Naturally, this feels rather frenetic and requires a calming influence. A calming influence is exactly what is delivered. Figs 4 to 6 on pages 6–7 illustrate these three variations in approach to treatment.

Apart from touching the different areas of the body to assess the quality and quantity of Ki within the Channels, the practitioner is likely to touch your belly area while you are lying on your back, with your permission of course. The interplay of Ki within the Channels and Organs can be assessed in this way.

With practice, the source of any disharmony can be narrowed down to two, or even one Channel. Each Channel has its corresponding area on the abdomen and the practitioner will assess these with either firm touch, light touch or by simply scanning the warmth and activity from each area using the palms, without actually making contact. Fig 42 illustrates the location of these areas.

The back of the torso also gives an area map of correspondences relating to internal Organs and Channels (see Fig 43). Imbalances reflected in the back areas can become visible to the trained eye, because when you scrutinize any example of the same thing often enough, you begin to see more detail and greater subtleties.

Some practitioners may also take a reading from your pulse, in exactly the same way as an acupuncturist would. There are six positions on each wrist, giving a total of twelve positions, all of which give an indication of the state of Ki within all the major Organs and functions of the body.

RECEIVING A SHIATSU
TREATMENT – PREPARATION

Having received the physical part of the health assessment, you will probably be lying down, although in some cases the assessment is done in a sitting position. You will have been asked to wear one layer of loose, comfortable clothing made of cotton or some other non-synthetic fibre. This is important because it is easier for the practitioner to feel the result of Ki imbalance through thin clothing. Why? Because contact with the skin tends to draw the attention of the mind onto the surface of the body instead of just below the surface where Ki flow is strongest. Synthetic fibres tend to interfere with your tactile sensitivity, whereas natural

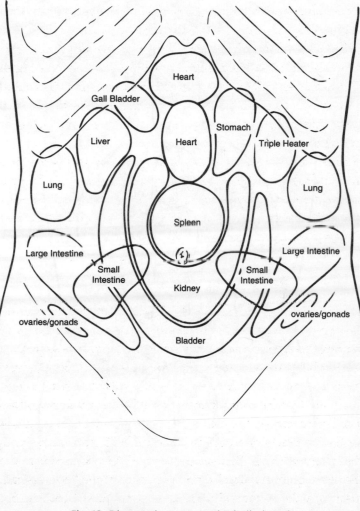

Fig 42: Diagnostic areas on the belly (Hara)

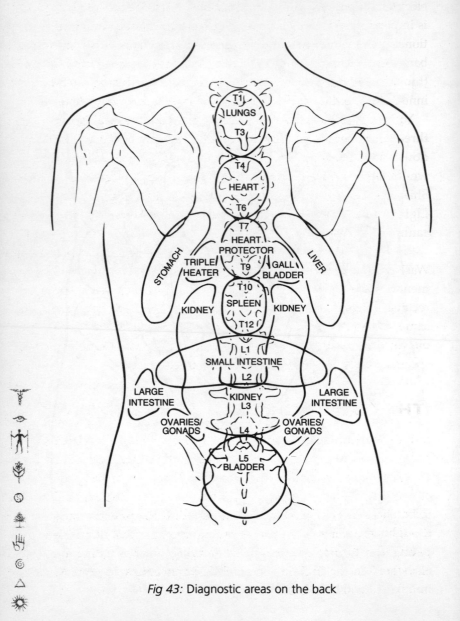

Fig 43: Diagnostic areas on the back

fibres are neutral. This may well be because of the increased static electricity produced within synthetic fibres. This layer of clothing is important, so if you go for a Shiatsu treatment and the practitioner prefers you to remove your clothes and wants to work on bare skin, please check his or her credentials again. Working through clothing has the added advantage of reducing sexual innuendoes, and it enables Shiatsu to be given almost anywhere.

You will also have been advised not to eat a large meal two to three hours before the treatment. This is simply because lying down with pressure applied to your torso after a full meal would feel too uncomfortable. If you have eaten a large meal, a Shiatsu may still be possible in a sitting or sidelying position. Light snacks beforehand are fine, as you should not feel you cannot relax due to hunger.

Ideally, Shiatsu feels much better if you can wash beforehand. Washing and changing into fresh clothing reserved for the treatment helps put you in the right frame of mind to 'open up' and receive touch. A sensitive practitioner will also have done the same. Obviously a wash and change may not always be possible for you, particularly if you are receiving a Shiatsu given spontaneously for something like an acute headache.

THE ESSENTIAL QUALITIES OF SHIATSU

Initially, the practitioner will place his or her hands upon your body and remain quite motionless in order to focus their mind as exclusively as possible upon you. This ensures a good connection with your body, enabling the subtle changes and imbalances in your vitality to be detected. If the practitioner's thoughts are somewhere else, dwelling upon the past or anticipating the future, or perhaps wondering what is going on elsewhere in the building, the subtle implications of your Ki imbalance will be missed.

To help you understand what the practitioner is doing, you should consider the essential qualities of Shiatsu, which are as follows:

Motivation	Support rather than force
Steadiness of breath	Correctly angled pressure
Keeping a low centre of gravity	Technical ability
	Continuity
Relaxation & comfort	Fluency
Empty mind	Empathy

MOTIVATION

If a person wants to make you feel better as much as you want to feel better, then you will have the foundation for a good healing relationship. Motivation to help others is a major requirement for becoming a Shiatsu Society registered practitioner.

STEADINESS OF BREATH

The rhythm of breathing is intimately connected to our thought processes. Consequently, if your mind is scattered and unfocused, the breath tends to be shallow and erratic. A focused mind is synonymous with steady, regular breathing. Conversely, to consciously breathe in a relaxed and steady rhythm helps focus the mind. Your practitioner will have invested a great deal of time in practising methods which promote steadiness of breath and consequent steady focusing of the mind. A focused mind is essential for detecting subtle energetic imbalances in your body. Meditation, Yoga and Tai Ji Quan are some of the methods many Shiatsu practitioners adopt to enhance the quality within themselves.

The practitioner will keep his or her centre of gravity as low as possible throughout the treatment to enhance maximum stability. Working from a stable base will allow the neck, shoulders and back muscles to relax. When the centre of gravity is too high, the postural muscles must overwork in order to maintain a steady position, resulting in early fatigue.

Your practitioner will ensure a low centre of gravity by;

- Keeping the hips spread open

- Keeping the belly relaxed to allow natural, deep breathing

- Keeping the mind focused on the breath as it expands and contracts the belly, so that their thoughts do not disperse

- Imagining the weight of their body to be accumulated on the undersurfaces, for example the undersurfaces of the forearms, lower surface of the belly and so on.

Once a low centre of gravity has been achieved and can be maintained, it is possible for all movement to originate from, and feel connected to, the lower belly. This enables weight to be used instead of force, enabling the body to remain totally relaxed. This in turn enables the practitioner to work without fatigue, and to concentrate his or her energy upon you, rather than upon their own discomfort, brought on by postural and muscular tension.

RELAXATION AND COMFORT

Steadiness of breath and keeping a low centre of gravity will enable your practitioner to remain relaxed. This is to the recipient's advantage because both tension and relaxation are infectious, especially where physical contact is involved. Better to be infected with relaxation than with tension. After all, to release tension and become relaxed is one of the reasons for receiving Shiatsu.

Relaxation and comfort are enhanced if Shiatsu can be done in quiet, pleasant, amenable surroundings. Also, wearing loose cotton rather than statically charged, clingy, artificial materials, avoiding flourescent lighting, and having an empty stomach without being ravenous will all add to comfort as well as promoting maximum energy levels.

EMPTY MIND

Shiatsu therapy requires both a developed intuition and the knowledge of how to put the theory into practice. Only by knowing something inside out can you then use it without intellectualizing about it. In practice, Shiatsu is much more about feelings than thinking. A practitioner cannot afford to be constantly thinking about what he or she should be feeling, because mental activity is also infectious. The consequent 'empty mind' of the practitioner will encourage the recipient's potentially restless mind to calm. Stress and tension are proportional to the restlessness of the mind. Likewise, relaxation and the potential to achieve optimum healing are proportional to the calmness of the mind.

SUPPORT RATHER THAN FORCE

If we push and poke at our fellow human beings, whether physically or mentally, we meet with resistance as they close up, fight back or withdraw. If we offer support they will feel secure, have trust and become receptive to our presence. This reality is particularly true in a Shiatsu situation.

The practitioner will offer you support in several ways. Firstly they will *assist* you to become healthier and more relaxed, rather than force relaxation upon you. Shiatsu practitioners see themselves as catalysts to support nature in restoring her balance, rather than as a means to force disease into submission.

Secondly, the practitioner will give the maximum physical support to ensure physical stability during the session. The most stable position for you is to lie flat in the prone or supine position, so that the floor is providing maximum support for your entire body. In this position, you can completely relax without fear of falling over, because you are already flat on the floor. In the sidelying position, you will be given a pillow to support your head, and your legs will be positioned in such a way to prevent your gradual collapse into prone.

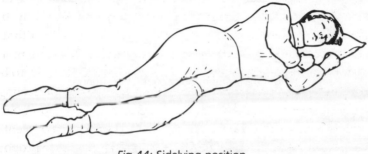

Fig 44: Sidelying position

Basically, the more vertical your position is for receiving Shiatsu, the more body contact you should receive to counteract the force of gravity. Shiatsu in the sitting position therefore requires maximum body contact to prevent collapse.

On the other hand, you may be one of those people who find too much support to be rather smothering, in which case the practitioner will support you more from arm's length, resulting in your having to take more responsibility for your own support. Part of the art of Shiatsu is to gauge how much support to give.

Thirdly, there is the supportive touch. Assuming you are not going to fall over when techniques are applied to you, you may st' eact defensively if you are pushed. That is why the

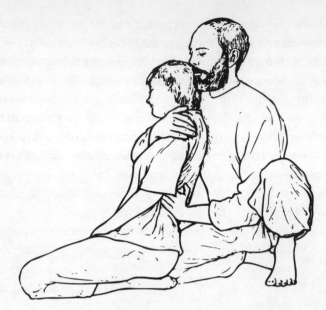

Fig 45: Maximum body contact in sitting

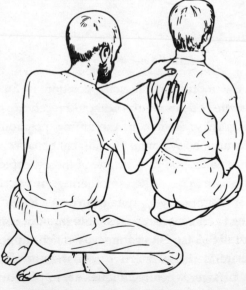

Fig 46: A more detached style of contact

PRINCIPLES OF SHIATSU

practitioner will *lean* into you rather than push, so that his or her pressure will be welcomed rather then repelled.

Finally, the fourth way the practitioner can be supportive to you is to be accessible enough to clarify any after-effects arising out of your Shiatsu session. It is possible to get a mild headache or a temporary worsening of symptoms after a treatment as the body re-adjusts itself to a healthier balance. If this should occur, a supportive word from your practitioner will put your mind at ease.

POSITIVE CONNECTION

Positive connection refers to both a positive rapport, and a positive physical touch. At your first session a good practitioner will seek to establish some area of common interest so that you can talk to each other as equals and on friendly terms, thereby establishing rapport.

On the physical level, positive connection means 'conscious' touch rather than mechanical touch. Conscious touch is where the mind of the practitioner is focused on the responses from your body as a result of his or her touch. Ki goes where the mind goes, so conscious touch enables Ki to be passed from the practitioner to you. Mechanical touch is touch applied with the mind elsewhere. This results in Ki neither being detected or projected. Only living beings have healing touch, which is why various machines and 'Shiatsu couches', which are claimed to give you a full body Shiatsu by mechanically prodding your pressure points at the flick of a switch, are of very limited value.

Even better than a 'conscious' hand on your body are two conscious hands on your body. With one point of contact, your mind is naturally drawn to that one point. With two points of contact, your mind is drawn to the connection between the two hands. This in effect means that a greater area of your body will feel involved in the treatment. Often the practitioner will create as many points of contact as possible by resting a knee or two against you so that your whole body feels enveloped by the treatment. This ensures that you feel fully supported, giving a much more nurturing feeling to the session.

CORRECTLY ANGLED PRESSURE

Stationary pressure angled at right angles to the surface of the body is the technique used to strengthen weak Ki, whereas moving, rocking, circling or pumping pressure is used to disperse blocked Ki. You are, no doubt, seeking Shiatsu because you feel under par, generally low in energy and possibly chronically ill, or because you feel uptight, frustrated or repressed in some way, as if you need to release some sort of 'valve' in order to relax. Low energy necessitates a treatment which is more tonifying. Feeling frustrated and blocked necessitates a treatment more dispersing in quality. However, behind every blockage there is an underlying weakness. This means that whether you are blocked up or depleted, your treatment will include an element of stationary holding Shiatsu. If you receive a treatment which is quite vigorous, including lots of rocking, stretching and pummelling, it means that a lot of unblocking of Ki was required. A treatment should never be 100 per cent vigorous, however, because everybody has a weakness which needs stationary holding pressure to tonify it.

TECHNICAL ABILITY, CONTINUITY AND FLUENCY

The skill of your practitioner is not a reflection of how many techniques he or she performs, but of their proficiency in delivering them well. Therefore, do not feel cheated if you find you are not being pulled and pressed about in a countless variety of ways. One well-connected, focused and relevant touch, held for anything up to five minutes, can have a tremendous effect upon your Ki.

A Shiatsu will have a fluent continuity about it. Often, as the receiver, you will never be quite sure exactly how you were moved from one position to another, or how the practitioner moved without you noticing. Moreover, Shiatsu is an art as much as a medicine. After a particularly good Shiatsu you feel you somehow 'hang together' better. This is tremendously fulfilling for both giver and receiver.

EMPATHY

As was mentioned previously, the Shiatsu practitioner invests a great deal of time in developing ways to increase sensitivity. Heightened sensitivity coupled with a genuine desire to help others results in the development of 'empathy'. Empathy is the fuel for intuition in Shiatsu. Individual practitioners will err towards the analytical or the intuitive. However, a really experienced practitioner will be able to deduce your imbalances from the Oriental Medical framework via the health assessment *and* intuitively feel where your problems lie. Empathy is another level of connection, and with optimum connection your Ki can be most profoundly benefited.

In short, all the essential elements of Shiatsu add up to provide you with a very rewarding and pleasurable experience, which will increase your body awareness and benefit your natural tendency towards optimum health.

WHO NEEDS SHIATSU?

Everybody needs Shiatsu because everybody benefits from as much balancing and strengthening of their vitality as possible. Nobody is in perfect harmony. However, you do not have to be ill to receive Shiatsu, although if you are, it can usually help in many ways. Even the most elementary Shiatsu is able to calm you if you are 'wound up', or loosen up your tense muscles and stiff joints, and strengthen your general level of vitality. Below are a few examples of circumstances when Shiatsu can be specifically beneficial.

SHIATSU HELPS ...

- increase energy levels
- increase body awareness
- relieve stress-related anxiety and tension
- induce very deep relaxation
- ease aches and pains
- boost the immune system
- treat common ailments
- increase flexibility
- heal sports and dance injuries
- stabilize emotional and psychological conditions
- relieve backache
- improve posture
- improve stamina
- improve digestion
- improve libido
- treat menstrual problems
- benefit a healthy pregnancy
- ease childbirth
- relieve headaches and migraines
- harmonize the body, mind and spirit.

Young, old, frail, strong ... it doesn't matter. If you can be touched, you can receive Shiatsu. However, there are certain circumstances where Shiatsu may be limited in its effectiveness, purely because touch is difficult and inappropriate. The following list highlights these situations.

- Acute fevers
  Most of us prefer to be left alone when we are aching and sweating from a fever.

- Contagious diseases
  It is not appropriate to touch someone with a disease that can be acquired through touch, for obvious reasons.

- Internal bleeding or blood clots
  If there is any suspicion of internal bleeding, Shiatsu should be avoided, because Shiatsu encourages an increase in blood flow. Blood clots are likely to break up or dislodge when pressed, or if blood flow is markedly increased. The dislodged clot or its debris could lodge in the heart or brain, cutting off the blood supply to these vital organs.

- Touch phobia
  If you hate being touched, then Shiatsu will be difficult for you. (On the other hand, Shiatsu might help you to learn to accept and enjoy touch.)

There are other situations where certain parts of the body must be avoided during a Shiatsu session. In these situations, the therapist will work on another area which, by association, benefits the area which cannot be touched. This makes sense if you accept that the body works as a functional whole; every part affects every other part at some level. No body part or function exists for its own sake. These situations include:

- Severe skin problems
  Psoriasis or eczema may be so severe that physical touch is too painful, and possibly damaging to the affected area of skin (although there is usually some part of the body that can be reached).

- Severe burns, bruises or swellings
Burns, bruises and swellings do not like pressure applied to them.

- Fracture sites and areas of acute muscle or ligament injury
Broken bones and torn ligaments should not be touched directly.

- Cuts, local inflammation and infections
Again, direct pressure would be agony.

- Twisted intestines
A twist in the intestines could easily become strangulated, thereby obstructing its own blood supply. It is conceivable that Shiatsu to the abdomen might strangulate an existing twist.

- Varicose veins
Direct pressure upon varicose veins is very painful and likely to cause damage to them. However, Shiatsu elsewhere can, to some extent, be of benefit in relieving the problem.

- During pregnancy
Shiatsu can be both very relaxing and very invigorating during pregnancy. However, certain pressure points can have a deleterious effect by increasing the risk of miscarriage.

  The lower leg is particularly rich in these contraindicated points. For this reason, if you are a 'mother to be', your Shiatsu therapist will avoid the lower leg altogether, except perhaps, for some gentle work on your feet (which can be exceptionally pleasant).

Shiatsu, by definition, requires actual physical contact. However, it is sometimes argued that techniques which use the heat radiating from the hands, but which do not make actual physical contact, can be considered supplementary Shiatsu techniques. These techniques are clearly not restricted in the contraindicated circumstances listed above. Radiating heat from the palms is called Hoshino therapy. This is not as difficult or mysterious as it sounds: just rub your hands briskly together and you can do it (Fig 48).

You can conclude from what I have said so far that Shiatsu can have a role in the management of most ailments. That role may often be very minor, or it may be very major. In many cases a different therapy will yield a faster and stronger result.

Shiatsu is definitely not the panacea sought after since the dawn of humankind. However, simply receiving human touch, rich in the Essential Qualities of Shiatsu, as described on pages 79–87, would fulfil a deep need in most of us. Humans are social creatures. We would all benefit greatly from sharing our Ki through touch. If everybody in the world knew, and was

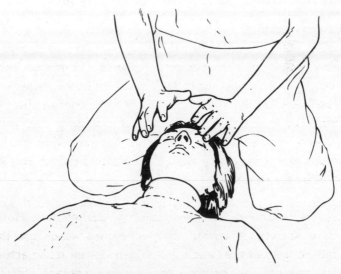

Fig 48: Radiating heat rather than touching

PRINCIPLES OF SHIATSU

prepared to give just enough general Shiatsu to keep each other's Ki channels open, then ill-health would be much less prevalent. Likewise, I am sure the world would be a much more peaceful place. Meanwhile, your local Shiatsu practitioner could help you in many ways.

TREATING SPECIFIC AILMENTS

Since most people suffer from various specific ailments at one time or another, it is useful to explore the effect of professional Shiatsu upon those ailments. However, always bear in mind that the treatment strategies described for each ailment relate to an archetypal situation. In practice, the actual treatment given and the Channels involved may vary. Shiatsu is designed to treat the person rather than the disease. Each person's disharmonies are unique, therefore each treatment will be unique.

Sometimes the effect of Shiatsu upon a person is to alleviate some of their symptoms or associated discomforts. An example of this level is the improvement in joint mobility achievable with Shiatsu in the management of disorders such as multiple sclerosis or hemiplegia. Sometimes Shiatsu can have a measurable effect at a deeper constitutional level. For example, it can improve the balance of hormonal secretions, thereby helping disorders resulting from hormonal imbalances, such as osteoporosis.

Every ailment described in this section is, of course, amenable to treatment from many different therapies. Where I have specifically mentioned other therapies, this indicates that I consider those therapies able to offer treatment as effectively as and, in some cases, more effectively than Shiatsu. However, in reality, it is the quality of the therapist which will determine success in helping you to overcome illness. An honest therapist will tell you if they feel somebody else can provide a more appropriate treatment.

If you are receiving treatment from a doctor and you wish to try Shiatsu as well, it is both wise and polite to discuss this with your doctor. Most doctors will be happy for you to receive some relaxing, vitality-boosting bodywork if considered appropriate. If your doctor has never heard of Shiatsu, lend him or her this book.

ACID STOMACH

Acid stomach can arise because of stress, overeating or eating the wrongs foods. Taking antacids will cause the stomach to produce more acid, making the problem worse in the long term. Therefore it is better to avoid them if possible.

Shiatsu given to disperse Ki in the Stomach Channel in the feet will cool the stomach and remove the sense of fullness. Shiatsu to the belly can also help.

ADDICTION

Addiction is a craving for, and dependence upon, a particular substance or 'drug' such as tobacco, alcohol, caffeine, heroin and so on. Drug dependence can be either primarily psychological or primarily physical. Psychological dependence results in craving or emotional distress when the drug is withdrawn. Physical dependence means the body has adapted to the presence of the drug, causing withdrawal symptoms when the drug is discontinued. Withdrawal syndrome is usually associated with severe physical and mental distress, including vomiting, trembling, cramps, confusion, anxiety, depression or, in the case of withdrawal from hard drugs, fits and coma.

Controlled withdrawal programmes are available in large hospitals and special centres. Some of these centres offer acupuncture, herbal medicine and counselling, which are especially effective during withdrawal. Shiatsu is also available in some centres and is of great value in helping to keep the withdrawal gradual and close to reality.

Shiatsu to improve and maintain vitality after the withdrawal process is complete may be more appropriate than acupuncture, due to the connotations associated with inserting needles. The general treatment aim will be to nurture the Kidney and Lung energy to boost Ki levels, strengthen willpower and cleanse the blood. Individual treatment will be tailored to deal with any of the numerous 'imbalances' left over from the residual effect of the substances taken. The Liver is commonly congested or damaged so the person will benefit from general dispersing or tonifying Shiatsu respectively. In addition, some calming techniques to the Heart Channel will help settle the mind.

AIDS

AIDS is a deficiency of the immune system thought to be due to infection with human immunodeficiency virus (HIV). However, AIDS (Acquired Immune Deficiency Syndrome) is not present in all those who are infected with HIV. It sometimes happens that people with a positive HIV diagnosis are found to have fought off the infection when re-tested at a later date. This suggests that giving more support to the immune system, and to one's psychological outlook, should result in more people throwing off the virus.

A combination of weight loss, fever and enlarged lymph nodes may appear in a person who has been infected with HIV, but does not actually have AIDS itself. These symptoms in combination are known as AIDS-related complex (ARC).

Shiatsu, along with Qi Gong (Ki-enhancing exercises) and Chinese Herbal medicine, has a role in helping to strengthen the immune system. Clinical practice has shown that projection of Ki into the Lung, Spleen and Triple Heater Channels has a positive effect upon the body's natural defences. However, Shiatsu reveals its strongest contribution to AIDS sufferers through its role of giving tactile support. The psychological support gained from receiving the supportive touch of Shiatsu is substantial.

ALLERGIES

Allergy means oversensitivity or intolerance of various substances such as pollen, milk, wheat gluten and so on. Most allergies are of a protein nature. The superficial treatment is to identify the offending substances and eliminate them from your life. However, Natural Medicine would consider allergies to reflect a weakness in the Liver's ability to process proteins, coupled with a weakness in the immune system. Tonifying Shiatsu to the Lungs, Triple Heater, Spleen and Kidney Channels will build up Ki, and therefore benefit the immune system. Dispersing style Shiatsu to the Liver and Gall Bladder Channels to help 'decongest' the Liver will often help, especially in combination with herbs and acupuncture. Both homoeopathy and dietary therapy can have good results with allergies.

ANAEMIA

Anaemia is a condition in which haemoglobin (the oxygen-carrying pigment in the red blood cells) is deficient. Anaemia will appear if the balance is upset between red cell production in the bone marrow and red cell destruction in the Spleen. It is most commonly the result of a deficiency of iron, which is an essential component of haemoglobin. However, anaemia can have numerous causes and is often itself a symptom of other illnesses.

The symptoms of anaemia result from a reduction in the capacity of the blood to carry oxygen. Mild anaemia can cause headaches, tiredness and lethargy. More severe conditions can cause breathing difficulties on exercise and dizziness due to reduced oxygen reaching the brain. Angina pectoris (see below) and palpitations may also occur. Some forms of anaemia result in jaundice, due to yellow pigment released by the rapid destruction of red cells. Iron deficiency anaemia occurs when the iron required for growth is not matched with sufficient intake of iron in the diet, or the ability of the digestive system to extract and absorb iron. Women are particularly subject to anaemia due to repeated loss of blood during menstruation.

In many cases Shiatsu can be of benefit by strengthening the Ki flow within the Spleen and Small Intestine Channels, thus aiding digestion, absorption of nutrients and the production of blood. In cases of heavy menstrual bleeding, Shiatsu can strengthen the Liver's function of 'storing the Blood'. However, it is essential that iron is replaced through foods containing iron, such as green vegetables and wholefoods. Herbal medicine (both Chinese and Western) is strongly recommended as there are many herbal formulas which contain iron and improve the absorption of iron.

ANGINA PECTORIS

Angina pectoris is chest pain caused by lack of oxygen to the heart muscle, usually resulting from poor blood supply due to coronary artery disease. Coronary artery disease arises from a narrowing of the arteries supplying the heart itself (i.e. the coronary arteries). This narrowing is caused by atherosclerosis (fat deposits on the walls of the arteries). Other causes of angina are: abnormal heart rhythms (arrhythmias); narrowing of the aortic valve in the heart (aortic stenosis); or intermittent spasms in the coronary arteries. Nicotine from smoking also increases atherosclerosis. Severe anaemia can also cause angina pectoris because of the reduced oxygen-carrying capacity of the blood. Other rare causes are thickening of the blood (polycythaemia) and excessive production of thyroid hormones.

Angina pectoris is aggravaged by any situation which makes the heart work harder, namely: during exercise, when under stress, in extremes of temperature, or following a heavy meal. The main symptom is chest pain with a sensation of pressure on the chest.

Nutritional counselling is usually useful in the management of angina, as is herbal medicine and homoeopathy. Shiatsu can be

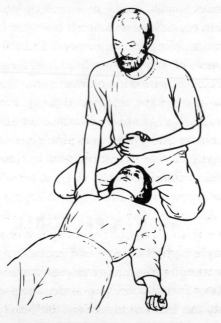

Fig 49: Calming the Heart Channel

useful to relax the blood vessels and ease the burden on the heart. The technique illustrated in Fig 49 shows the practitioner calming the Heart Channel. This can be useful during an acute attack.

ANKYLOSING SPONDYLITIS

This is a disease which starts with pain and stiffness in the lower back and hips, resulting from inflammation of the sacro-iliac joint (joint between the spine and pelvis) and the joints between the vertebrae of the spine. These symptoms are worse in the early morning and after resting. It is of unknown cause, more common in men than in women, and tends to run in families. Inflammation in the spine eventually leads to some permanent stiffness and limitation of movement, plus varying degrees of spinal curvature (kyphosis). Breathing may be restricted, causing pain in the chest due to stiffening of the joints between the spine and the ribs.

There is no known treatment which can cure ankylosing spondylitis, but the symptoms may be reduced by deep dispersing style Shiatsu or massage to the back muscles, and heat applied to the back. (Note: heat would not be used where there was active inflammation.) Heat could be applied using palm heat (Hoshino therapy), compresses made from hot ginger, or moxa (see page 162). The most important treatment is exercises to keep the back muscles strong, increase breathing efficiency and to improve posture. Swimming and Yoga are particularly appropriate. An adjunct to Shiatsu technique called *Sotai* is also beneficial (see page 163). Sufferers might consider the Alexander Technique for maintaining and improving posture.

The inflammatory process becomes less active with age so if treated consistently, with plenty of appropriate exercise, ankylosing spondylitis leaves only minor deformity and loss of movement.

ANOREXIA NERVOSA

This is a disorder mainly affecting young women, centred around wilful avoidance of food and intense fear of being fat. It is characterized by severe weight loss causing disruption in the balance of sex hormones. This often leads to cessation of menstrual periods (amenorrhoea).

There is much controversy over the cause of anorexia. Underlying causes are difficult to identify. The most successful line of approach is a long course of psychotherapy, which must be continued even after the symptoms have disappeared. Since many sufferers appear to have a distorted image of themselves, Shiatsu can be of use insofar as it can stimulate, through touch, a different awareness and perspective of one's body. Shiatsu to the Spleen, Kidney, Lung and Heart Channels may help to reduce the anxiety associated with this condition.

ANXIETY

Anxiety can range from mild apprehension to extreme fear. It is only a problem if it is extreme enough to inhibit thought and disrupt normal everyday activities. Sufferers usually have a fear that something bad is going to happen to them. The common physical symptoms are palpitations, throbbing or stabbing pain in the chest, a feeling of tightness in the chest and an inability to take in enough air. There is often a tendency to sigh or even hyperventilate (over-breathe). These chest symptoms can in turn create spasms in the neck, back pain, headaches due to muscular tensions and an inability to relax. Digestive disorders are also usually present, in particular, nausea and dryness of the mouth.

Orthodox medicine attributes anxiety to psychological causes. In particular it forms theories based either on the fear of losing loved objects, or on learned behavioural conditioning whereby drive to increase performance becomes a deeply habitual anxiety.

Oriental Medicine would see the excessive worry and pensiveness of anxiety as indicative of a Spleen imbalance. The Spleen imbalance would in turn affect the Kidneys, therefore exacerbating fears and phobias. Conversely, it could be the Kidneys which are ultimately affecting the Spleen; a classic 'chicken or egg' situation. The symptoms of chest pain, tightness in the chest and inability to take in enough air are caused by the Kidneys failing in their function to pull Ki down from the Lungs. The Lung involvement gives rise to the classic anxiety symptoms of feeling cut off from the world, or from oneself (a

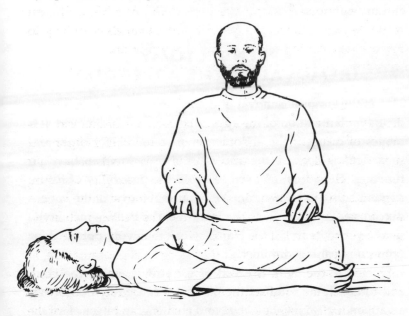

Fig 50: A point on the breastbone (Directing Vessel 17) and another in the lower abdomen (Directing Vessel 6) are held simultaneously to 'connect' the Lungs and the Kidneys.

PRINCIPLES OF SHIATSU

reflection of the Lungs' failure to fulfil their function of maintaining a sense of 'boundary').

Shiatsu treatment given with lots of physical contact and support is excellent for rebalancing the Spleen and strengthening the Kidneys. A specific technique to help the Kidneys pull Ki down from the Lungs and thus facilitate relaxed rhythmic breathing is illustrated in Fig 50.

Shiatsu to the Heart Channel in the arms would be of value for its calming effect upon the mind.

All the acute symptoms of stiff neck, backache and headache can be relieved with general dispersing style Shiatsu to the back and neck.

Some counselling or psychotherapy is indicated for most chronic sufferers.

APPENDECTOMY (REMOVAL OF THE APPENDIX)

This is the surgical removal of the appendix following appendicitis (inflammation of the appendix). Often it is removed as a matter of course if the abdomen is operated on for other reasons. This is because the appendix is considered to have no function. Thus, it is removed to avoid the possibility of future appendicitis. I have mentioned it because removal of the appendix substantially weakens the Hara (i.e. the belly, which is the seat of your vitality). If the Hara is weak then your potential for optimum health is diminished.

Shiatsu to the belly is excellent for strengthening the Hara and thus helping to offset the weakness caused by not having an appendix. Tai Ji Quan, Yoga and challenging physical activity all strengthen the Hara. If you do not want to do any of those things, then regular Shiatsu would be very helpful.

ARTERIOSCLEROSIS

This is a blanket term for various disorders that cause thickening and loss of elasticity of artery walls. The most common type is atherosclerosis, which is described under angina pectoris. For treatment of atherosclerosis see angina pectoris (page 97).

ARTHRITIS

Arthritis means inflammation of a joint. There are several different types, but all are characterized by pain, stiffness and usually swelling. Arthritis may involve one joint or many, and may vary in severity from a mild ache and stiffness to severe pain with joint deformity.

The most common type is osteoarthritis (also called osteoarthrosis) which results from wear and tear to the joint. Diet, metabolic and genetic factors may contribute to its onset. It most commonly troubles older people.

The most severe type is rheumatoid arthritis, caused by the body's immune system acting against joints, damaging them and their surrounding tissues. It most commonly affects the hands, wrist, arms and feet, involving greater heat and swelling than osteoarthritis.

Gout is a type of arthritis which is caused by an accumulation around joints of uric acid crystals (one of the body's waste products) causing inflammation. It is usually due to slightly malfunctioning Kidneys, or excessive strain on the Kidneys from over-consumption of acidic foods and drink (e.g. meat, alcohol).

Alterations to diet will help to ease many of the symptoms in most types of arthritis. Herbal medicine, acupuncture and homoeopathy can all be very effective. Osteopathy, chiropractic, Shiatsu, physiotherapy and the Alexander Technique can be of value in osteoarthritis by maximizing the correct alignment of joints and improving posture. This would have the effect of reducing further wear and tear upon the joints.

For many sufferers of rheumatoid arthritis there would appear to be a substantial psychological/emotional factor contributing to its onset. For those people, psychotherapy may provide some answers. Where there is acute rheumatoid arthritis affecting many joints, the role of Shiatsu is limited, as the inflamed joints, and much of the rest of the body, are simply too painful to be touched. In the acute situation, the Shiatsu practitioner can use techniques which strengthen the Kidneys, and can also smooth the flow of Ki by working around joints (not on them) and by calming or dispersing the Liver and Gall Bladder Channels. The Kidneys and Gall Bladder (in the Oriental Medical sense) are invariably implemented in all types of arthritis.

In short, for acute inflammatory arthritic conditions I would recommend you first try acupuncture with herbs, or homoeopathy. In less acute cases I would, in addition, advocate Shiatsu or other forms of bodywork which work on maintaining mobility in the joints. However, great care must be taken by any therapist dealing with joints in the neck in people with rheumatoid arthritis. This is because the neck area can become very fragile in these circumstances.

ASTHMA

Bronchial asthma is where spasm of the small airways in the lungs (bronchioles) results in recurrent breathlessness and wheezing. Attacks can be precipitated by stress or anxiety, or triggered by a wide variety of stimuli, such as dust, exercise, infection, pollen or allergy to a particular food. A cough may develop due to bronchial inflammation causing an increase in the production of phlegm.

A severe attack will cause rapid heartbeat and sweating with increasing breathlessness and wheezing which prevents the sufferer from lying down or sleeping. Very severe attacks can be fatal.

Asthma is very common, affecting 5 per cent of the adult population and 10 per cent of children. The symptoms are most commonly controlled by inhaling a drug such as Salbutamol which relaxes the airways.

Oriental Medicine explains asthma as a weakness of the Lungs and Kidneys, coupled with an acute invasion of Wind and Cold (see Causes of Disease, page 66). Shiatsu treatment is aimed at relaxing and strengthening the Lungs and strengthening the Kidneys. A specific Shiatsu technique which accomplishes this is illustrated on page 101 under 'anxiety'. You may be able to make Lung Ki descend and stop an attack yourself by circling your thumb into a point called Lung 6, seven thumb widths above the wrist crease on the inside of the forearm, in line with the thumb. After an attack, the Shiatsu practitioner will work down the Bladder Channel on the back, particularly concentrating on tonifying the Lung and Kidney transporting points.

Herbs, acupuncture, homoeopathy and aromatherapy all have a lot to offer asthma sufferers. However, in severe acute attacks, a doctor should always be consulted. Another type of asthma called cardiac asthma results from heart failure or reduced pumping efficiency of the heart. This also requires close supervision by a doctor.

BACK PAIN

Back pain can result from numerous mechanical causes, for example muscle tears, ligament strains, damage to a spinal facet joint or prolapse of an invertebral disc ('slipped disc'). Other causes include osteoarthritis, ankylosing spondylitis, coccydynia (pain at the base of the spine usually resulting from falling on the coccyx) or cancer in the spine.

Shiatsu, like osteopathy and chiropractic, is excellent for dealing with back pain resulting from mechanical causes. However, many causes of backache are the result of weakness in the Kidneys. Oriental Medicine attributes the strength of the spinal column, and of bones generally, to the Kidneys. Consequently, even problems in the vertebral joints may ultimately be due to Kidney weakness. Shiatsu is one of the most relevant therapies for strengthening the Kidneys and is especially effective in combination with the appropriate Chinese herbs.

Backache frequently accompanies a local blockage of Ki in the Channels which run through the back, buttocks and hips. The Kidney and Bladder Channels along with the Small Intestine and Large Intestine Channel extensions are common culprits. Shiatsu technique is very efficient at unblocking these Channels.

Weak abdominal muscles predispose one to general fatigue and pain in the lower back. Abdominal strengthening exercises are therefore very important. Most physiotherapists can recommend the most effective abdominal/back exercises.

My recommendations are that if you have severe back pain of unknown cause, or due to structural misalignment, you should see a chiropractor or osteopath. If structural realignment fails to cure the problem, then Shiatsu may well be successful on an energetic level. Shiatsu corrective exercises (Sotai) are very effective where there is muscular imbalance distorting the posture. If you think the problem is Kidney weakness, consider seeing someone who practises Chinese herbal medicine to supplement your Shiatsu treatments (herbs work well with acupuncture or Shiatsu). General back aches may result from poor posture, in which case both the Alexander Technique or the Feldenkrais method are excellent.

BRONCHITIS

Bronchitis is inflammation of the mucous membranes of the bronchial tubes (airways) with short, rapid, wheezy breathing, infection and a productive cough. Chronic bronchitis has very intractable and persistent symptoms which distinguish it from asthma, in which wheezing and breathlessness vary in severity from hour to hour throughout the day. Oriental medicine regards bronchitis as an imbalance in water metabolism and weakness in the Lungs.

Shiatsu treatment would strengthen the Lungs, open the chest and help regulate water metabolism. There are many specific Shiatsu techniques which can be directly applied to the rib cage for the purpose of clearing phlegm from the lungs (see Fig 51). There are also many herbs which are of benefit.

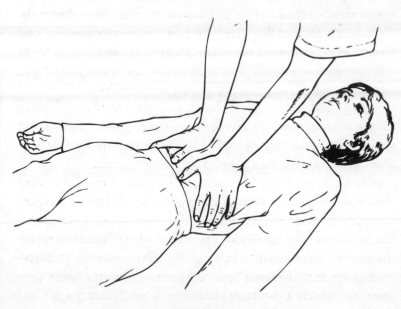

Fig 51: Clearing phlegm from the lungs

PRINCIPLES OF SHIATSU

Bronchitis often co-exists with emphysema, in which the air sacs in the lungs become distended. Together, these conditions are called chronic obstructive lung disorder (COLD) or chronic obstructive airways disease (COAD). However, the treatment principles are the same as for chronic bronchitis.

BRUISING

Bruising is caused by leakage of blood from damaged capillaries causing discoloration beneath the skin. It usually results from a blow or injury. Ice-cold compresses applied for 10 minutes usually halt its expansion. Homoeopathy works wonders with speed of recovery. Shiatsu is of little use in alleviating acute bruising. In fact, massage or Shiatsu can make it worse. However, Shiatsu focused on the Spleen and Heart Channels may help those with a tendency to bruise severely from relatively minor knocks. This is because the Spleen's energy is responsible for holding the Blood in the blood vessels. The Heart's energy controls the strength of blood vessels.

BULIMIA

This is a disorder which involves gross overeating followed by self-induced vomiting. Its causes and treatment are very similar to anorexia nervosa (see page 100).

BURNS

Shiatsu is not directly relevant for burns. Western medicine, or the use of certain essential oils as prescribed by a well-qualified aromatherapist, are better options. However, Shiatsu could help alleviate the shock associated with burns (see Shock, page 151).

Cancer is defined as any group of diseases in which symptoms result from the unrestricted growth of cells in one or more of the body organs or tissues. The outcome of the disease depends upon the location of the tumour, at what stage it is treated and the determination of the sufferer to recover.

The role of Shiatsu in this situation is not to 'treat' the cancer, but to help raise the overall vitality of the person. With more vitality, we are in a better position to cope with whatever befalls us.

If you have cancer and decide to receive Shiatsu, do so for the purpose of strengthening your Ki rather than expecting Shiatsu to cure the cancer. Shiatsu cannot claim to do that. Also inform your doctor of your intention to receive Shiatsu. Whatever treatment is applied should always be in cooperation with a doctor. For one thing, they are the only ones who can record its level of success.

The method of Shiatsu will be light, supportive touch rather than strong technique upon specific pressure points. Judge whether or not Shiatsu is of any use to you by seeing if it makes you feel any better either physically or psychologically.

CARPAL TUNNEL SYNDROME

This is a condition where a ligament at the front of the wrist puts pressure on the median nerve which runs underneath it. This pressure interferes with nerve impulses carried by the median nerve to the hand, causing numbness or tingling, and weakness in the thumb. It occurs most commonly in women during menopause or during pregnancy, in those who have just started using oral contraceptives or who suffer from premenstrual syndrome. Clearly therefore, it is often connected to female hormonal imbalance. Men or women who suffer from rheumatoid arthritis may also suffer due to tissue inflammation and swelling around the wrist.

Shiatsu, herbs, acupuncture, reflexology and homoeopathy can all help rebalance the hormonal system. In Oriental Medical terms this means regulating Ki and Blood in the Internal Organs, especially the Liver, Spleen and Kidneys. Dispersing style Shiatsu on the hands, arm and shoulder will help 'smooth' the flow of Ki, Blood and Body Fluids through the wrist.

CATARRH

See Nasal Congestion, page 140.

CEREBRAL PALSY

This is a general term for damage to a child's developing brain causing either spastic paralysis (abnormal stiffness and contraction of muscles); athetosis (involuntary writhing movements); or ataxia (loss of coordination and balance). Most cases occur before or at birth. The severity can vary from slight to complete disability. Mental retardation occurs in about 75 per cent of cases.

Cerebral palsy is not curable as such, but much can be done to improve muscular control and balance. Physiotherapists are the people most qualified and able to do this. However, many Shiatsu therapists have found that very patient, focused and supportive Shiatsu can considerably reduce muscular spasms. For parents of children with cerebral palsy, learning some basic Shiatsu would be useful and rewarding.

CHILDBIRTH

Childbirth is clearly not an illness, but nevertheless can be an incredibly painful and exhausting experience. It may be very helpful if there is someone present during labour who can give Shiatsu. Women in labour often find the supportive 'distraction' of Shiatsu to be a godsend. Working on the neck, shoulders and lower back often helps reduce pain considerably. However, some women do not want to be touched *at all* during labour, in which case reserve Shiatsu for the days after the birth. Then it will be highly appreciated.

The ideal person to give Shiatsu during labour is the husband or a very close friend. Not all husbands and close friends are Shiatsu therapists, but a short course in basic technique could substantially increase their usefulness. (For information on courses, see resources section on page 176).

For Shiatsu during pregnancy, see page 146.

COMMON COLD

The common cold is a viral infection causing inflammation of the mucous membranes leading to the copious production of mucus. Most commonly, the mucous membranes of the nasal passages and sinuses are affected, although the ears, eyes and throat can also be involved. It is not curable as such, meaning that once you have a cold, it must go through a particular cycle before the symptoms subside. However, there is some evidence that large doses of vitamin C can help prevent a cold, or hasten its end.

Regular Shiatsu would contribute to keeping the immune system strong and thus help prevent colds. Once you have a cold, Shiatsu applied to the face can do a lot to help decongest the nasal passages and sinuses (see Sinusitis, page 152). Dispersing style Shiatsu to the Lung area on the upper back and the Lung Channel in the lower forearm would help eliminate Wind and Cold (see Causes of Disease, page 66) and strengthen the Lungs.

CONSTIPATION

Constipation is the difficult and/or infrequent passing of hard, dry faeces. According to Western medicine, this may be due to excessive water absorption from the bowel, spasms or lack of tone in the muscles of the bowel wall, a low fibre diet, a habitual neglect of the desire to go, or a bowel obstruction such as a tumour.

The Oriental Medical explanation of a short-term constipation may be excessive internal Heat from emotional problems or hot spicy food. A long-term problem may arise from weak Ki and Blood.

Shiatsu is an excellent treatment for constipation because it can be administered directly to the abdomen. It is through the abdomen and lower back that Ki can best be strengthened. This is because a close connection can be made to the 'Gate of

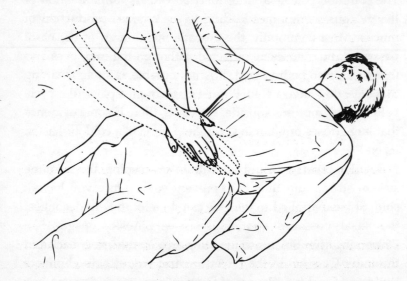

Fig 52: Wave rocking technique on the belly

Vitality' (the source of bodily Ki). The strength of Blood is largely to do with the efficiency of the intestines, which can also be tonified directly, through pressure on the abdomen. There are also several specific pressure points on the belly and elsewhere which alleviate constipation. Symptomatically, a deep wave-like action applied by the hands to the belly can really shift things.

Another good tip: eat an apple before going to bed, and drink a glass of cold water upon waking up. If this fails, try also eating a tablespoon of honey first thing in the morning.

Avoid laxatives as far as possible; they will only make things worse in the long term. If your regular bowel movement pattern changes or if your constipation occurs suddenly, consult your doctor.

CONVALESCENCE

If you are resting up, recovering from an illness or operation, this is a great time to receive some good tonifying Shiatsu. Convalescence really means allowing space for your Ki to strengthen, and strengthening Ki is a speciality of Shiatsu. Therefore, the more Shiatsu you can get, the better.

CORONARY ARTERY DISEASE

See Angina Pectoris (page 97) and Atherosclerosis (page 103).

CRAMP

Cramp is painful spasms in a muscle often occurring during or immediately after exercise. Western medicine explains this as a buildup of lactic acid and other chemicals in the muscles as a result of increased muscular activity. It can also be due to an overactive nerve reflex affecting blood circulation within the muscle. Cramp in resting muscles is usually due to loss of sodium salts through sweating in very hot weather or during prolonged exercise.

From the viewpoint of Oriental Medicine, cramps result from local stagnation and/or deficiency of Ki and Blood. Shiatsu techniques can regulate this. Tonifying Shiatsu to specific pressure points on the Bladder Channel behind the knee and calf muscle can tonify Ki and Blood. This works much better in tandem with appropriate nourishing herbs if the cramping is recurrent.

Shiatsu can give immediate relief by stretching the muscles concerned, and/or by dispersing the Liver and Gall Bladder Channels and specific pressure points. If you get writer's cramp, you can disperse this yourself by circling your thumb firmly in the middle of the web between the thumb and index finger, close to the joint.

DEPRESSION

Depression can show itself as a general loss of interest in life, hopelessness, pensiveness and feelings of sadness. It can bring on fatigue, poor appetite, shortness of breath and sleeplessness. There may be obvious causes for being depressed, such as the loss of a close relative, or one may become depressed for no obvious reason. Either way, Shiatsu can be of some help by using techniques on the Heart Channel to calm the Mind, and other techniques to invigorate the circulation of Ki and Blood in the Heart, which will help lift depression.

In many cases there may be an obvious role for counselling and psychotherapy. Bach flower remedies are also helpful.

DERMATITIS

Dermatitis is a blanket term for inflammatory skin conditions (see Eczema).

DIABETES MELLITUS

There are two types of diabetes mellitus. The most severe form is where no insulin is produced because the insulin-producing cells of the pancreas are destroyed, probably as a result of a viral infection damaging the immune system. This type is more likely to appear in people under 35 years old. The other type is where insulin is produced, but not enough to meet the body's needs. This type is of gradual onset, and is more likely to affect people over 40.

Lack of insulin causes the level of sugar in the blood to remain abnormally high, causing excessive thirst, frequent copious urination, hunger, fatigue and sometimes loss of weight. Diabetes also upsets fat metabolism and accelerates the degeneration of small blood vessels.

Diabetes is controlled by insulin injections and/or regulation of diet. However, it is extremely difficult to 'cure', and can lead to an endless list of possible complications, such as damage to the retina, damage to nerve fibres, kidney damage, cardiovascular disorders and so on.

If some insulin is still being produced by the pancreas, in some cases Shiatsu treatment aimed at strengthening the Spleen and Kidneys can reduce the severity of symptoms. Reflexology has also helped in a few cases that I know of, as has Chinese herbal medicine.

DIARRHOEA

Diarrhoea is looseness of the bowels, resulting from malabsorption of food and water, or the creation of excess fluid and mucus from the bowel lining. It may be due to diet, nervousness, or infection, and if severe is often treated with antibiotics or kaolin and morphine. In terms of Oriental Medicine, it is a lack of warming Ki (Yang Ki – see page 35) in the Spleen, Stomach and Kidney, or an excessive intake of watery 'Damp' foods.

The Shiatsu practitioner would strengthen the Kidneys (the source of warming Yang Ki) in the lower back, and work on several points on the Bladder Channel in the lower thoracic and lumbar regions; which regulates the Spleen's function of eliminating Damp and generally regulating the movement of water in the lower body. In many cases, the therapist would use moxa to these points (see moxa, page 162).

If diarrhoea is severe, especially in young children, see a doctor straight away. This is because serious dehydration can occur, and can be fatal in babies and young children.

DIVERTICULOSIS

Diverticulosis is a condition of the colon where small sacs or pouches protrude externally from the walls of the lower colon. These sores, called diverticula, are thought to be caused by pressure forcing the lining of the colon through areas of weakness in the wall. If the diverticula become inflamed, the condition becomes diverticulitis, which is much more serious.

Shiatsu cannot do anything to specifically treat diverticulosis. However, this condition is often accompanied by muscle spasms and cramps in the colon. The general principles of treatment listed under 'cramp' would apply here to give some symptomatic relief (see Cramp, page 113).

Down's Syndrome is a common type of mental handicap accompanied by characteristic physical features. It is caused by an abnormality in the chromosomes affecting the development of the fetus. It is more common in babies of mothers who give birth when over the age of 40. It cannot be cured, but a lot can be done to improve the child's life by providing an affectionate and supportive home environment. General Shiatsu can contribute at this level. A parent can learn some basic Shiatsu and share it with the child, who usually finds it immensely enjoyable. The child also often finds it enjoyable to copy the giver and do it back to them.

Cranial osteopathy given at a very early age has proven to be very beneficial in many cases. The use of nutritional supplements also appears to help. Certainly, good nutrition with well-prescribed supplements for mothers during pregnancy may well reduce the likelihood of Down's Syndrome manifesting in the child.

DRUG DEPENDENCE

See Addiction, page 94.

EARACHE

This is extremely common, especially in childhood. Causes may arise from infection, congenital defect, ear wax, boils, vertebral misalignment in the neck, or a side-effect of drugs. However if none of these causes seem to be present, the earache may be a manifestation of Ki blockage within the Gall Bladder or Triple Heater Channels. Shiatsu aimed at dispersing these Channel blockages would help. This would involve Shiatsu to the side and back of the head.

If vertebral misalignment is suspected, then treatment from an osteopath or chiropractor would be the best option.

ECZEMA

Eczema is a term used to describe a variety of inflammatory skin conditions. It is characterized by itching and scaling of skin. The cause is not known in many cases, although it is sometimes due to allergy. Western medicine will usually treat it with corticosteroid creams. If it is severe and affecting large areas of the body surface, then Shiatsu is of little value, simply because you cannot apply pressure to such areas. In less severe situations, and where there is a clear allergenic factor, the same principle of treatment can be applied as described under 'Allergy' (see page 96). For eczema it is well worth taking a prescription of Chinese herbs and looking closely at the diet.

EMPHYSEMA

See Bronchitis, page 107.

EYE SORENESS

Sore eyes include painful, red, swollen, itching and bloodshot eyes. There may be symptoms of external irritations, infection, sinusitis or a cold. Reading in poor light when excessively tired can also cause it.

Shiatsu can help through local pressure point techniques to the face, head and eye sockets. Dispersing techniques to the Liver and Gall Bladder Channels in the feet cool and brighten the eyes and move stagnant Ki from the eyes.

FACIAL PALSY

Facial palsy is a weakness of the facial muscle due to injury or inflammation of the facial nerve. The most common type is called Bell's palsy. Facial palsy often clears up spontaneously. Facial exercises are an essential element in regaining normal facial expression. Shiatsu to the face can help relieve the pain and may facilitate recovery. Acupuncture can have very good results.

FAINTING

Fainting is defined as 'temporary loss of consciousness due to insufficient oxygen reaching the brain'. It may result from low blood pressure, stress, shock, fear or lack of oxygen causing slowing of the heartbeat via overstimulation of the vagus nerve, which supplies the heart. This type of fainting is known as vaso-vagal attack. Fainting may also be due to irregularity of the heartbeat preventing adequate blood flow to the brain.

From a Shiatsu therapist's perspective, fainting represents a necessity to counteract a deficiency of blood circulation. Various first aid acupressure techniques could be used, one of which is to firmly press the area between the nose and upper lip with the thumbnail until the person comes round. The other hand would be resting on top of the person's head, which in itself helps to restore consciousness. You could try this yourself if somebody faints, in addition to normal first aid procedures. However, if they do not completely recover within a minute or two, or if it happens again, get the person to hospital immediately.

FATIGUE

Fatigue can be due to depression, anxiety and other emotional factors, or it can be due to physical overwork. Either way, these causes add up to a deficiency of Ki. Tonifying deficient Ki is the main contribution of Shiatsu along with the dispersal of blocked Ki. Shiatsu to the lower back, abdomen and Kidney Channels, plus the use of some specifically invigorating pressure points, will help considerably. Chinese and Western herbs, acupuncture, reflexology and relevant nutritional advice are all very useful. Fatigue can also result from postural and structural imbalances, in which case osteopathy and chiropractic can help. Both Yoga and Qi Gong will boost one's level of energy and therefore combat fatigue.

FEVER

Most fevers are the result of invasion by pathogenic factors, namely bacterial or viral infections. Fevers may also be symptomatic of dehydration or overactive thyroid glands.

During a fever, Shiatsu is best avoided because one usually needs to be left alone to 'sweat it out'. Between fevers, if they are recurrent, certain pressure points and Shiatsu techniques can be used to help strengthen the Lungs and thus invigorate the body's protective Ki. Likewise, a general Shiatsu programme to strengthen the immune system is a good idea. I would recommend Chinese herbal medicine or homoeopathy as additional measures.

FIBROSITIS

Fibrositis refers to pain and stiffness in muscles, probably resulting from stagnation of Ki and blood circulation due to poor posture or sitting in cramped positions. It seems to be aggravated by tension, anxiety and cold damp weather. Although it is common in middle-aged and elderly people, many doctors dismiss it because they fail to find any measurable reason for the symptoms. The neck, back, shoulders, chest, buttocks and knees are commonly affected.

Shiatsu treatment is aimed at moving the stagnant Ki and boosting the circulation of blood in the affected areas. This simply requires locally administered vigorous dispersing techniques. Subsequent tonification of the Kidney and Spleen Channels, and dispersal of the Liver and Gall Bladder Channels usually helps to minimize further episodes.

FLAT FEET

This condition is where the ligaments and muscles supporting the arches of the feet have weakened or failed to develop. If it develops in adulthood, a programme of exercises to strengthen these muscles and ligaments can help. A physiotherapist or chiropodist would recommend the appropriate exercises. Shiatsu to tonify the Kidney, Liver and Spleen can enhance the effectiveness of corrective exercises. This is because the Kidney and Spleen Channels support the arches. The Spleen supports and 'holds things up' in general within the body. The Liver nourishes ligaments, including those supporting the arches.

FLU (INFLUENZA)

See Fever, page 120.

FRACTURES

A fracture is a 'broken bone'. The fracture site should be kept well clear of Shiatsu. However, after the bones have been set and healing has begun, other areas of the body can receive general Shiatsu to improve blood circulation and Ki flow, thereby increasing energy and nourishment to the site of injury.

FROZEN SHOULDER

Frozen shoulder is most common amongst middle-aged people. It is restriction of movement in the shoulder accompanied by pain. It results from inflammation of the capsular ligament around the joint. This inflammation develops for no known reason. In some cases it follows an injury to the shoulder, angina pectoris, chronic bronchitis or a stroke. Recovery is usually slow, irrespective of which treatment is given. Shiatsu can often give good results by tonifying local deficiencies of Ki within Channels passing close to the shoulder; in particular the Heart and Heart Protector Channels, plus the Stomach, Spleen and Kidney Channel extensions. Gentle mobilizing movements for the shoulder also help, plus a general full body Shiatsu.

GLANDULAR FEVER

This is more correctly called 'infectious mononucleosis' which is an acute viral infection causing swollen lymph glands, particularly in the neck. The main symptom is a severe sore throat. Young adolescents are the most likely to suffer, as it affects those who encounter the virus for the first time, at a time when their immune system is most vigorous. In severe cases mild liver damage may occur, resulting in jaundice.

Most patients recover after a few weeks without medicinal treatment. Subsequent rest is required to allow the body's immune system to destroy the virus. For a further two or three months, the patient will feel sleepy, lacking in energy and often depressed. It is during the period of rest and recovery that Shiatsu can be of immense benefit in tonifying the immune system. Projection of Ki into the Lung, Spleen and Triple Heater Channels has a positive effect, as does patient tonification of the Kidneys. However, those who have suffered glandular fever

usually exhibit slightly deficient Ki in the Liver and Gall
Bladder Channels for years afterwards. Regular Shiatsu can
benefit this.

GOLFER'S ELBOW

See Tennis Elbow, page 155.

HAEMORRHOIDS

Haemorrhoids or 'piles' are swollen veins occurring close to
the anal opening (external haemorrhoids) or high up in the
anal canal (internal haemorrhoids). They can also protrude
outside the anus (prolapsing haemorrhoids). The usual cause
is internal pressure on the veins from straining to pass hard
faeces. They also commonly occur during pregnancy. Those
who eat highly refined foods lacking in dietary fibre can be frequently affected.

Shiatsu can help in mild recurrent cases by tonifying the
Spleen Channel which helps prevent all types of prolapses.
Anal problems in general are helped by treating the Bladder
and Kidney Channels. Treating the Large Intestine Channel in
the legs will help relieve any associated constipation, as will
dispersing the Liver Channel in some cases. Tonification of the
Heart Channel may help strengthen the veins in the long term.
In the short term, herbal poultices applied to the area will help.

HAY FEVER

Hay fever is an allergy to pollen, house dust, or other airborne
substances. The treatment principles are the same as for allergies in general (see Allergies, page 96).

HEADACHES

Headaches result from altered circulation in the head due to physical, emotional or dietary causes. Imbalances in the Liver and Gall Bladder Channels cause migraine headaches and headaches on the side of the head; Stomach and digestive imbalances cause headaches in the forehead.

The Shiatsu practitioner's approach would be to disperse the stagnant Ki in the head and to regulate Ki in the Organs by applying specific techniques to points on the head, neck and feet. In addition, Shiatsu to the Stomach Channel in the leg will help clear frontal headaches; while Shiatsu to the Liver and Gall Bladder Channels in the head and legs will clear headaches on the side of the head. Headaches occasionally accompany constipation, and thus clear up when correct bowel movements are returned. Shiatsu to the Large Intestine Channel and abdomen can help in such situations (see Constipation, page 112).

Cranial osteopathy and herbal medicine can also cure headaches in many instances.

If the headache is particularly severe and intractable, or accompanied by blurred vision, consult a doctor immediately.

HEART ATTACK

If someone nearby has a myocardial infarction, which is commonly called a heart attack, please do not take them to a Shiatsu practitioner, reflexologist or anybody else other than a *doctor*. Call an ambulance immediately.

If you personally have had an attack before, or think you are a candidate for getting one, then Shiatsu may be of some help in strengthening the Heart and Heart Protector, whilst reducing stress and tension. Stress is a factor which considerably increases the risk of heart attack if the other causative factors are present. Attention to diet, smoking and drinking habits are extremely important.

HEMIPLEGIA

Hemiplegia is a term used to describe weakness or paralysis on one side of the body. It occurs as a consequence of damage to the nerve tracts in the opposite side of the brain. Usual causes are strokes, head injury, brain tumour, meningitis or in some cases, multiple sclerosis. One or more of the following sites may be affected: the arm, leg, part of the torso or the face.

Treatment is aimed at restoring function to the affected parts of the body. Physiotherapists and occupational therapists are by far the most experienced people in dealing with this. Shiatsu can be effective in helping to restore awareness and movement to the affected side of the body. Severe hemiplegic patients tend to lose awareness of their affected parts to the extent that they 'forget' those parts even exist. Since Ki goes where the mind goes, Shiatsu is an ideal catalyst for putting both Ki and the consciousness back into those forgotten areas.

Hemiplegia can be either 'spastic hemiplegia' which means the muscles are held in spasm and therefore 'stiff', or 'flaccid hemiplegia', where the muscles are limp and wasted. Flaccid hemiplegia requires very patient holding and tonifying of the Channels within the affected areas. Spastic hemiplegia requires careful stretching and light dispersing techniques to the affected Channels, plus general calming Shiatsu. Both types require the affected limbs to be moved frequently and in graded stages, to maintain and improve joint mobility.

Ultimately, the success of any treatment depends upon the extent of the brain damage and the motivation of the patient.

HERNIA

There are many types of hernia, most of which consist of a protrusion of the intestine through a weak area in the abdominal wall. The most common type is an inguinal hernia, in which part of the intestine bulges through the inguinal canal in the groin. Some hernias can be pushed back. Those that cannot be pushed back usually require surgery.

The Shiatsu therapist can help some mild hernias by tonifying the Channels associated with the Organs located in the area of the hernia. Thus, for inguinal hernias, the Large Intestine and Small Intestine Channels would be treated. For all hernias, the Spleen may also be treated, due to its role in 'holding things up' in the body.

Another type of hernia is hiatus hernia, in which the Stomach protrudes through the diaphragm into the chest. Here, Shiatsu can ease the discomfort by applying certain stretches to the ribcage.

HERPES

The herpes simplex virus may cause painful blister-like rashes on the genitals, lips, mouth or face. It is highly contagious, but does not necessarily manifest its symptoms unless the person is under stress, anxious, depleted in energy or has a weakened immune system. Shiatsu can help to minimize the appearance of symptoms by boosting Ki, and completely relaxing the recipient to reduce the effect of stress and generally boost the immune system. Treatment to the Spleen and Liver Channels often helps a little. Homoeopathy is excellent for tackling the infection at a deeper level. Chinese herbs can also be very helpful.

HICCUPS

Hiccups (also spelt Hiccoughs) are sudden, involuntary contractions of the diaphragm. Shiatsu can stop most hiccups instantly by applying pressure to the Back Transporting Points in the lower thoracic region. If this fails, simultaneous pressure to the outermost edge of each shoulder usually succeeds.

HIGH BLOOD PRESSURE

Abnormally high blood pressure is called *hypertension*. It is extremely common, affecting around 15–20 per cent of the population in developed countries. It can be caused by disorders of the kidneys or adrenal glands, complications in pregnancy, congenital heart defects, and the use of certain drugs. It can also be brought on by smoking, excess alcohol, sedentary lifestyle and prolonged stress.

Shiatsu treatment to the Heart and Heart Protector Channels can help relax the constricted artery walls. General calming Shiatsu acts on the parasympathetic nervous system, which will de-stress the recipient, and can also relax the artery walls. If the Kidneys or adrenals are involved, then Shiatsu to the Kidneys may help. Both Yoga and Qi Gong also considerably reduce hypertension. However, the true cure is a radical moderation in smoking, drinking, alcohol, dietary excess and stress factors.

HYPERGLYCAEMIA

This is an abnormally high level of sugar (glucose) in the blood. It is a feature of inadequately controlled diabetes mellitus (see page 115).

HYPOCHONDRIASIS

Hypochondriacs are people who worry excessively about their health. It can be a complication of other psychological disorders. In some cases it may be helped by Shiatsu or Acupuncture focused mainly upon rebalancing the Spleen and Stomach, as these Organs relate to pensiveness and worry. However, most chronic sufferers require the skills of a psychotherapist. Bach flower remedies can be very effective for many people.

HYPOGLYCAEMIA

This is an abnormally low level of sugar (glucose) in the blood. It is a feature of diabetes mellitus or can occur from an excess intake of alcohol. Treatment will be as for diabetes mellitus (see page 115).

IMMUNODEFICIENCY DISORDERS

Any disorder which is the result of failure of the immune system's defences to fight infections and tumours is called an immunodeficient disorder. HIV and AIDS are well-known examples. Overuse of drugs and congenital defects are commonly implicated. Oriental Medicine attributes the cause to weakness of Defensive Ki and Nourishing Ki. Shiatsu, by its very nature, strengthens Ki. In particular, tonification of the Kidney, Spleen, Lung, Large Intestine and Triple Heater Channels can be very helpful, because these Channels and Organs all contribute significantly to the strength of Defensive and Nourishing Ki. Specific herbs and good diet are very powerful tonics for the immune system, as are Qi Gong and Yoga.

IMPOTENCE

Impotence is the inability to achieve or sustain an erection. Most cases are symptomatic of stress, anxiety, depression or other psychological factors. However, physical factors can be the cause. For example, it may occur as a reaction to certain drugs, hormonal influences, damage to the spinal cord, or excessive alcohol. It becomes more common in men as they get older.

If the cause is psychological in origin, then counselling or psychotherapy is recommended. Shiatsu can help lift anxiety or depression, and reduce the effects of stress.

If the cause is an hormonal imbalance, calming followed by tonification of the Kidney and Bladder Channels may help. If restricted circulation is the problem, causing failure to erect, the Liver Channel would receive dispersing techniques whilst the Heart and Heart Protector Channels are tonified, to move the Blood. Lack of sex drive may be helped by Shiatsu to the Spleen and Stomach Channels (to stimulate an 'appetite' for sex and a desire to procreate) and the Kidney Channel (the kidneys provide will, drive and impetus).

INCONTINENCE

Incontinence is the inability to withhold urine. It may be due to many possible factors, such as injury, stress, obstruction such as enlarged prostate gland, prolapse of the uterus or vagina, mental impairment, or weakness of the pelvic muscles.

Shiatsu can help where the cause is weakness of the pelvic muscles, by applying an adjunct to Shiatsu known as Sotai corrective exercises (see page 163). Tonification of the Kidneys should help because they control the opening and closing of the urethra. Tonifying Shiatsu to the Liver and Spleen Channels in the legs can also help. Acupuncture is very effective, and it is worth doing some good old pelvic floor exercises.

INDIGESTION

Apart from cases where it is a symptom of some more serious disorder, indigestion arises from overeating, or eating too rapidly, both of which cause food to stagnate in the stomach. There are various pressure points in the abdomen whose specific actions, when dispersed, are to move the food stagnation and increase circulation in the stomach and intestines. The Stomach and Spleen Channels would also be treated, as they directly influence digestion.

Reflexology is often effective, as are specific herb teas. Food combining, as advocated in the Hay Diet, has helped many sufferers from chronic indigestion.

INFECTIOUS DISEASES

Shiatsu is not an appropriate therapy to treat infectious diseases. Western medicine, and in some cases Chinese or Western herbs, are called for. However, a person who has a tendency to develop repeated infectious diseases may benefit from Shiatsu which is given between infections, and aimed at strengthening the immune system (see page 128).

INFERTILITY

Infertility is the inability to produce offspring. Male infertility is usually due to a partial or total failure to produce sperms, or malformation of the sperms. It may also result from failure to produce sperms with sufficient lifespan to reach the egg. Smoking, certain drugs and general toxicity can reduce the sperm count. In some cases, sexually transmitted diseases can damage the spermatic ducts.

Female infertility usually results from failure to ovulate. Hormonal imbalances, stress, congenital defects, fibroids in the uterus, ovarian cysts or tumours may be the cause. Also, blocked fallopian tubes may prevent the sperm from reaching the egg. The other possible factor is failure to conceive if the cervical mucus produces antibodies that kill the male sperm.

Shiatsu, acupuncture and/or Chinese herbs can help male or female infertility if the problem is failure to produce sufficient, or correctly formed sperm or ova. This would be considered a weakness of constitutional Ki or 'Essence' (see page 8). Strong nurturing and tonification of the Kidneys would be required, possibly supplemented by techniques to help the Liver move Blood to the reproductive organs. Please note that it could take a long time to achieve results. If the cause is an hormonal imbalance, it could be treated in the same way. If it is purely stress-related, then general Shiatsu will be of great benefit. Hormone replacement therapy is often successful for infertile women. It is advisable to receive a medical examination to check for causes due to physical blockages, such as cysts or tumours.

INSOMNIA

Insomnia is difficulty in sleeping. It can be a by-product of many physical and psychological disorders. Oriental Medicine sees it as a deficiency of Heart energy and Blood, due to emotional problems or an unbalanced lifestyle. The Heart-Ki and Blood keep the Mind anchored and calm; therefore, deficiency in either will cause the Mind to be overactive. This will be exacerbated at night if the body's cooling functions are weak (expressed as Yin deficiency in Oriental Medicine). Feeling too hot at night, with a restless mind, thus amounts to insomnia. A congested Liver may also cause sleeplessness.

Shiatsu treatment similar to that given for depression may help (see page 114). If caused by a congested Liver, dispersal of the Liver Channel will be given. Acupuncture combined with Chinese herbs can be very successful for insomnia. Insomnia due to a traumatic incident or situation playing upon the mind may require psychological counselling.

IRRITABLE BOWEL SYNDROME

This is the most common disorder of the intestine and is twice as common in women as in men. It is a disturbance of the muscular contractions which create bowel movements, causing intermittent cramp-like pain, abdominal swelling, a sense of incomplete bowel evacuation, and excessive wind. It is aggravated by food. Sufferers are usually in good health apart from suffering the symptoms described.

The cause is not clearly understood, but emotional stress and anxiety will exacerbate the condition. Shiatsu can help balance these emotions (see Anxiety, page 100 and Depression, page 114).

Like constipation, this condition requires strengthening of the Ki and Blood, and balancing of the colon function. Alternate tonification and dispersal of the Bladder Channel in the lower lumbar region can help relieve the severity of the symptoms.

JET LAG

Jet lag occurs when air travel across different time zones causes your body and mind to experience a longer or shorter day. This sudden anomaly in time upsets your natural body rhythm, causing fatigue, poor memory, disorientation and a disturbance in your sleep cycle.

Receiving general Shiatsu after a flight is superb for minimizing jet lag. The very core of Shiatsu is its balancing effect upon the body's energies, hormones and rhythms; the very essence of jet lag is its unbalancing effect upon the body's energies, hormones and rhythms. If you travel a lot and frequently suffer from jet lag, I can guarantee Shiatsu will change your life.

JOINT INJURIES

Any joint can be injured due to a fall, blow or an over-zealously performed exercise. Most injuries will be of the ligaments supporting the joints or involve a fracture. The treatment of acute ligament injuries is described on page 134 and fractures on page 121. As the joint recovers, Ki and Blood needs to be moved into and around the joint to minimize stiffness. Dispersing style Shiatsu to numerous pressure points around the affected joint will achieve this. Specific stretches can also be used. The Shiatsu therapist will know when the joint injury is old enough to receive direct Shiatsu by feeling the quality of Ki within the local pressure points. Treating these points too soon will cause acute pain. (See Ligament Sprain below).

LEUKORRHOEA

Leukorrhoea refers to abnormally heavy, white vaginal discharge with inflammation and itching in the vaginal area. The cause is bacterial or fungal infection. It is characterized by poor circulation and coldness in the pubic area. Shiatsu techniques to the Liver Channel, plus stretching the legs can help improve circulation to the genitalia. Additionally, treatment of the Small Intestine and Triple Heater Channels will help most female reproductive disorders.

LIGAMENT SPRAIN

Ligaments are bands of strong, fibrous tissue which bind bones together and stabilize joints. They are sometimes damaged by injury or inappropriate exercise. A ligament injury takes longer to recover than a muscle injury because ligaments have no direct blood supply. In contrast, muscles have a very extensive blood supply.

Shiatsu can slightly improve the speed of recovery by tonifying the Channels which pass through the injury site. Techniques are *not* applied directly on the sprain, but either side of the injury and any accompanying muscle spasm. The effect of this is to increase blood circulation to the tissues surrounding the ligament. It is by diffusion of blood from surrounding tissues that ligaments receive their nutrients. Shiatsu and Sotai corrective exercises to align the associated joint accurately will also speed up recovery.

Shiatsu, acupuncture or herbal medicine to balance the functions of the Liver can help strengthen the ligaments in general and thus reduce the risk of sprain. Herbal poultices and homoeopathy also have a lot to offer here.

LORDOSIS

Lordosis is an exaggerated concave curvature of the lumbar spine. It can result from weak abdominal muscles, weak Kidneys or over-contraction of certain deep muscles connecting the inner pelvis to the lumbar vertebrae. Wearing high-heeled shoes can cause it by tilting the pelvis forward, forcing the spinal curves to become exaggerated. Certain types of dance training which over-emphasize backward bends can also result in lordosis.

Shiatsu to tonify the Kidneys, strengthen the belly, relax the deep lumbar/pelvic muscles (especially Iliopsoas), and

rebalance the general posture can be very effective. Shiatsu is
even more effective if combined with a programme of Sotai
exercises. Also, many people with lordosis can be, and have
been, helped with the Alexander Technique.

LOW BLOOD PRESSURE

Blood pressure which is below 'normal' is only a problem if it
is causing discomfort, such as fatigue, dizziness, insomnia,
headaches, palpitations, poor circulation, lack of concentration
or any other symptoms. General tonifying Shiatsu can help over
a period of months. Specific Shiatsu techniques to deal with the
associated symptoms are helpful in the short term. Medical
herbalism, acupuncture and homoeopathy may also be of
benefit.

LUMBAGO

See Backache, page 105.

M.E.

M.E. stands for Myalgic Encephalomyelitis. It is also known
as post-viral fatigue syndrome and epidemic neuromyasthenia.
Main symptoms are muscle fatigue on exertion, general ma-
laise, depression and inability to concentrate. Sleep disturbances,
dizziness and nausea are common features. It may follow an
infection in the respiratory or digestive tract, with accompanying
headaches and fever. However, the precise cause is unknown. A
viral infection resulting in damage to the immune system would
seem to be the most likely explanation. There are three times
more women sufferers than men. Many sufferers also suffer from
the fungal infection known as candidiasis or thrush.

M.E. usually clears up eventually, but may persist for many years, especially if exacerbated by stress. Shiatsu therapists can teach sufferers to cope more easily with stress and directly reduce their stress-related physical tensions (see Stress, page 154). In addition, Shiatsu can play a positive role in strengthening the immune system (see Immunodeficiency Disorders, page 128). Acupuncture, herbs and nutritional therapy can help in many cases.

MENOPAUSE

Menopause is the natural cessation of menstruation that women experience as they reach between 45 and 55 years of age, as a result of reduced production of the female sex hormones. Symptoms such as hot flushes, vaginal irritation, tiredness, insomnia, irritability and night sweats are common. Oriental Medicine explains these symptoms as an imbalance in the Kidneys' cooling energy (Yin) leading to imbalance of Ki and Blood in the Heart, Spleen and Liver.

Shiatsu can help by tonifying certain points on the Kidney Channel which nourish the cooling Yin, and by dispersing points on the Heart Channel which move Blood Stagnation, stop flushes and night sweats, and calm the Mind.

MENSTRUAL DISORDERS

The reproductive system is influenced by internal body rhythms regulated by the hormonal system and blood circulation. These can be easily disturbed by physical, emotional and nutritional factors. Imbalances can manifest as menstrual pain, heavy menstruation, irregular menstruation or pre-menstrual syndrome.

In Oriental Medicine, exposure to cold, excess cold food, and weakness or stagnation of Ki and Blood can cause these imbalances. The Shiatsu practitioner will use techniques to regulate Ki and Blood to the internal organs, especially the Liver (which stores the Blood and smoothes Ki flow) and the Spleen (which discourages haemorrhage by holding Blood in the blood vessels).

Menstrual pain can be relieved by treating the Stomach and Small Intestine Channels, plus points on the Liver and Spleen Channels. For pain and dizziness after the period, the practitioner will tonify the points on the Bladder Channel in the mid and lower back. Shiatsu to the lower lumbar and sacral area will help to improve menstrual regularity. Heavy menstruation is dealt with by Shiatsu to the feet, big toe and lower belly. Premenstrual syndrome will cause irritability, depression, breast distension, nausea and lower abdominal bloating. The practitioner will smooth the flow of Ki by dispersing blocked Ki in the Liver Channel, and calm the mind by calming the Heart and Spleen Channels. Acupuncture, herbal medicine and homoeopathy are all potentially effective therapies for menstrual disorders.

MIGRAINE

See Headaches, page 124.

MULTIPLE SCLEROSIS

Multiple sclerosis is a disease of the brain and spinal cord of unknown cause, but which is thought to be an auto-immune disorder. It differs markedly in severity amongst sufferers. It affects young adults and is slightly more common in women. The actual changes in the nervous system appear to be due to some action in the body which dissolves or breaks up patches of the protective covering of the nerve sheaths. The symptoms vary according to which parts of the nervous system are affected. Feelings of heaviness in the limbs, tingling, numbness or feelings of constriction can result from spinal cord damage. Clumsiness, muscle weakness, slurred speech, blurred or double vision, fatigue, vertigo and numbness may result from damage in the brain.

The distinguishing characteristic of M.S. (multiple sclerosis) is its unpredictable improvements and remissions, followed by sudden relapses. Some people are mildly affected, with long remissions, and occasional recurrence of minor symptoms. Others are severely disabled within a year or two of developing the disease. Stress, over-strenuous exercise and too much exposure to direct sunlight can exacerbate or trigger the symptoms. Dietary modifications help some sufferers, particularly the inclusion of sunflower seeds and evening primrose oil.

Shiatsu during remissions can help reduce stress and boost the immune system, thus potentially reducing the risk or severity of symptoms recurring. When symptoms are present, Shiatsu with Sotai corrective exercises can help strengthen the muscles. Other forms of less subtle muscle strengthening can actually cause an increase in the severity of symptoms. In my experience, most sufferers from M.S. have marked imbalances in their Spleen and Heart Protector Channels. Shiatsu to these Channels can often relieve the severity of many associated symptoms. Sometimes, careful tonification of the Bladder Channel down either side of the spine can radically increase the person's vitality and mobility for a few days. Sometimes you can do all of these treatments and nothing changes whatsoever. Such is the unpredictable nature of multiple sclerosis.

MUSCLE STIFFNESS

If you overdo an exercise to which you are unaccustomed, the blood circulation through the muscles involved will prove inadequate to flush away the waste products from the cells and tissues produced during the exercise. Regular exercise gradually increases the efficiency of local blood circulation, so that post-exercise stiffness becomes less severe.

Shiatsu is of tremendous help in invigorating the Ki and blood circulation, both locally and generally. A specific method of stretching the muscle fibres at right angles to the direction in which they lie helps squeeze these waste products out. Fig 53 illustrates this principle of 'cross fibre' stretching applied to the thigh.

Appropriate essential oils such as Lavender or Rosemary applied by a good aromatherapist will also give good results. Note that muscle stiffness will be markedly reduced if a thorough warm up before exercise, and a 'warm down' after exercise, are carried out.

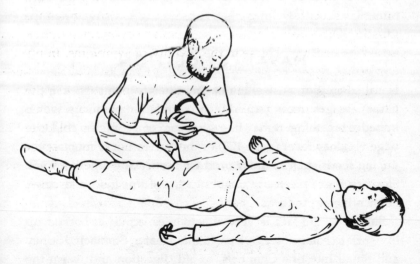

Fig 53: Cross fibre stretching to the thigh

MUSCLE STRAIN

Muscle strain is the tearing of some muscle fibres within a muscle belly, resulting from a sudden or extreme movement. The pain and swelling is due to engorgement of blood from the broken capillaries within the torn muscle fibres. Shiatsu or massage should never be applied to an acute strain because it will increase blood circulation and make the swelling and pain worse. Apart from brief applications of ice to the injury, muscle strains should be left alone and allowed to rest for two or three days. After a few days, when the internal bleeding between the muscle fibres has stopped and congealed, Shiatsu or massage can be applied to the surrounding tissues in order to increase the blood circulation. This will facilitate the removal of debris and waste products from the injury and allow incoming blood to bring nutrients for repair. Homoeopathic first aid preparations administered at or shortly after the time of injury will help minimize shock, swelling and pain.

NASAL CONGESTION

Nasal congestion is swelling of the mucous membranes in the nasal passages, accompanied by accumulation of mucus, which impedes breathing. It may be a symptom of a common cold (see page 111), hay fever (page 123) or the overeating of mucus-producing foods such as dairy products; especially where a weak Stomach and Spleen are unable to transform food and drink efficiently.

Shiatsu to the face is very effective, especially if backed up by work to balance the Spleen, Triple Heater, Stomach, Kidney and Small Intestine Channels, to aid digestion and warm the body.

NAUSEA

Nausea is the sensation of needing to vomit. Its treatment is the same as for 'indigestion' (see page 130). You can help relieve nausea and motion sickness by holding firm pressure into a point called Heart Protector 6, or 'Inner Gate'. This point lies in the middle of the lower forearm, two thumb widths above the wrist crease on the palm side. Shiatsu to the feet can also help.

NEUROSIS

Neurosis is a term ascribed to fluctuating intensities of emotional and psychological feelings. Neurotic disorders include forms of anxiety, depression, obsession and many other emotions. The difference between neurosis and psychosis is that the neurotic person is fully aware of his or her psychological state. They remain in touch with reality.

Most sufferers from neurosis will benefit from the feelings of connection and support offered by Shiatsu. The Five Element model of Oriental Medicine attributes certain emotional imbalances to each organ (see page 59). By observing which emotion is predominantly within a neurosis, the Shiatsu practitioner can deduce which organs need rebalancing. For example, anxiety and obsession with fear involves the Kidneys, whereas overthinking involves the Spleen. In practice, it requires a bit more than merely treating the Channel associated with the prevailing emotion. However, a very experienced practitioner can use their understanding of Oriental Medicine to good effect. Some practitioners may use Bach flower remedies to supplement the treatment.

OSTEOARTHRITIS

See Arthritis, page 103.

OSTEOPOROSIS

Osteoporosis is a condition in which the density of bone diminishes, causing the bones to weaken, thus rendering them more liable to fracture. It is a natural result of ageing, but occurs more commonly and to a greater degree in women after the menopause. This is because their ovaries no longer produce sex hormones which help maintain bone density. A calcium-deficient diet, hormonal disorders, prolonged immobility or prolonged treatment with corticosteroid drugs can also create the disorder.

Hormone replacement therapy has significantly reduced the number of fractures caused by osteoporosis in women after the menopause. Shiatsu can help by focusing techniques upon the Kidney and Bladder Channels, thus helping to rebalance hormonal activity. The treatment principles for menopause are relevant for osteoporosis (see page 136).

OVARIAN CYST

Ovarian cysts are very common. They are fluid-filled enlargements of ovarian follicles (egg-producing part in the ovary). They vary in size from that of a pea to that of a football, although most are smaller than a golf ball. They often cause no symptoms although some women experience menstrual irregularities or pain during intercourse. Most cysts go away on their own; in fact many women have had them without realizing. Some require surgical removal.

Shiatsu can help prevent their recurrence, or speed their disappearance by helping to rebalance the hormonal system. This is achieved by tonifying the Kidney and Bladder Channels. Also, by strengthening the Spleen's function of transforming food and drink into body tissue, less residual waste products would be available to stagnate as fluid and mucus around the ovaries. Shiatsu, in combination with Chinese herbal medicine and a carefully tailored nutritional programme, is definitely the best way to keep those cysts at bay.

PALPITATIONS

Palpitations are the sensation of rapid and forceful heartbeat. They are often felt after strenuous exercise or in any situation where the heart is working hard, such as tense or scary situations, or when anxious. They may occur at rest, in which case they are usually the result of a high intake of alcohol or caffeine, or smoking. They may also be caused by irregularities of the heartbeat or overactivity of the thyroid gland. Palpitations are not necessarily problematic in themselves, unless they are very severe, causing chest pain, dizziness and breathlessness. Such extreme cases should be dealt with by a doctor.

Shiatsu to the belly and solar plexus is highly beneficial in reducing palpitations. It also helps to give calming techniques to the Heart and Heart Protector Channels. Palpitations may arise from retention of food in the stomach, or after eating excessive sugar. In these situations, balancing of the Stomach and Spleen Channels would help.

PANIC ATTACKS

Panic attacks occur during periods of acute anxiety. They usually last for only a few minutes and are rarely associated with any serious physical disorder. Many panic attacks are associated with various phobias, especially fear of dying or fear of losing one's sense of reality.

Psychotherapy has a definite role to play for many sufferers. However, Shiatsu is very useful due to its extremely efficient ability to induce total relaxation and a sense of 'grounding'. Shiatsu can also be of help on a deeper level by employing techniques to calm the mind and strengthen the will. Thus, the Heart Channel would be calmed and the Kidney Channel would be tonified. Also, the Stomach Channel may require calming or dispersing when the mind is disturbed.

One of the essential qualities of a good Shiatsu therapist is steadiness of breath. This ensures their mind is very calm and focused, giving a very grounded demeanour. These states of mind are infectious, so that the 'cool' Shiatsu practitioner may well stop a panic attack just by being present.

Bach Flower remedies, Yoga, Qi Gong and counselling can also be of benefit.

PARALYSIS

Paralysis is loss of voluntary movement resulting from the inability to contract affected muscles. Paralysis affecting one half of the body is called hemiplegia. Paralysis of both legs and part of the trunk is called paraplegia. Quadriplegia is paralysis of all four limbs and the trunk. Paralysis of varying degrees may be caused by a variety of injuries to or disorders of the brain, spinal cord or peripheral nerves. It may also result from a muscle disorder. Treatment principles are similar to those described for hemiplegia on page 125. For facial paralysis see page 119.

PARANOIA

Those suffering from paranoia experience the delusion of being persecuted or that certain people or events are especially connected to them. They rarely recognize these traits within themselves. Brain damage, alcohol and drug abuse, schizophrenia and other personality disorders are precipitating factors. Acute paranoia may also develop in people who have been radically 'uprooted' from their environment, such as refugees, immigrants or people who have suddenly become estranged from their families and friends.

Psychological counselling is the obvious treatment to try initially. The Shiatsu therapist might see the problem as based upon fear resulting from becoming uprooted, plus overthinking, with a sense of being ungrounded and unsupported. Rebalancing of the Kidney energy for counteracting fear, the Spleen energy for grounding and reducing overthinking, plus calming of the Heart and Heart Protector Channels to 'anchor' the mind is a likely treatment strategy. Fullness of the Stomach Channel often accompanies an agitated mind and may therefore also need calming. A Shiatsu style which is very supportive, yet highly focused, is the ideal medium for success with paranoia. Bach flower remedies and homoeopathy are also relevant for this condition.

PHOBIA

A phobia is a persistent, irrational fear of a particular object or situation. For example, agoraphobia is the fear of public places. The treatment principles from a Shiatsu perspective are very similar to those applied to paranoia.

There is a very simple, yet subtle technique for offsetting emotional disturbances. It requires that the practitioner lightly touch the forehead just above the eyebrows, in line with the centre of each eye. He or she then relaxes and focuses upon the pulses that are felt there. Your Shiatsu therapist might use this technique for any situation where the thoughts or emotions are scattered or confused. It inhibits subjective thought whilst promoting objective thought. Consequently, it enables the recipient to think more rationally for a few minutes.

PILES

Piles is the common name for haemorrhoids (see page 123).

P.M.T. (PRE-MENSTRUAL TENSION)

See Menstrual Disorders, page 136.

POLIO

Polio is an abbreviation for poliomyelitis. It is a virus which can attack the brain and spinal cord and lead to extreme paralysis involving the legs and lower trunk. Often, only one leg is affected. However, such damage only occurs in a very small percentage of cases. Over 90 per cent of people who pick up the virus suffer nothing more than a sore throat and slight fever.

Most of those who suffer some resultant paralysis make a full recovery with the help of physiotherapy to help retrain and improve muscle function. Of those that do not, less than 25 per cent are left with severe disability. Shiatsu can have a role in helping to minimize 'postpolio' deterioration; a situation where nerve weakness and pain recurs in some of the muscles, years after a partial recovery has been made. The treatment principles are to increase blood circulation and Ki to the affected limbs by strengthening the Liver, Kidney, Heart and Spleen Channels. In cases of near recovery after prolonged paralysis, Sotai corrective exercises can help correct musculo-skeletal imbalances.

PREGNANCY

Pregnancy is not an illness, but one of the most natural of phenomena, occurring throughout the animal kingdom. As such it is not necessary to 'treat' it, and much better to leave it alone if all is going smoothly. For this reason I would recommend you avoid Shiatsu sessions which emphasize deep sustained pressure on specific pressure points. However, pregnancy may give rise to local aches and pains resulting from changes to posture and to one's centre of gravity. Dispersing style Shiatsu to the spaces between the ribs and to the shoulder blades is extremely helpful for eliminating pain and stiffness commonly experienced in those areas. Neck stretches and techniques to ease lower backache are also particularly helpful. Because of the existence of 'the bump', your therapist would treat you in the sidelying or sitting position. As regards treatment during labour and after childbirth, see Childbirth, page 110.

PROLAPSED UTERUS

A prolapsed uterus means the uterus has descended from its natural position down into the vagina. Shiatsu cannot do anything to reverse the situation, but it can help prevent it happening. Therefore if you are a likely candidate for a prolapse, the therapist would focus attention on tonifying the Spleen Channel. One of the Spleen's functions, by definition of Oriental Medicine, is to hold up and support the Internal Organs. Shiatsu given to the belly area, plus Sotai corrective exercises for the pelvic region, would also be extremely beneficial.

PROSTATE PROBLEMS

For reasons unknown to Western Medicine, the prostate gland can swell and press against the urinary tube, interfering with urination. If severe, the usual treatment is removal of the prostate. When giving Shiatsu, we usually find those with prostate problems have a Liver Channel which feels empty (kyo) and a Kidney Channel which feels empty, but with an apparent, superficial fullness. The Liver Channel supplies the prostate with its energy to function, whereas the Kidney furnishes it with 'Essence' to make semen.

If the problem is not too severe, Shiatsu may well be able to stop it getting worse. In this situation the Kidney Channel usually requires mild dispersing techniques, followed by strong tonification of the Liver and Gall Bladder Channels. After a few treatments, the Kidney Channel would then benefit from gentle tonification, as would the Bladder and Spleen Channels. Chinese herbal medicine would be an ideal supplement to these treatments.

Regular pelvic floor exercises are effective in helping both to treat and to prevent prostate problems.

PSORIASIS

Psoriasis is an inflammatory skin condition which can cover a very extensive area of the body's skin surface. For this reason, it is not amenable to Shiatsu treatment, other than the hands off, palm healing techniques. However, if the skin inflammation disappears as a result of other treatment, such as Western medicine, homoeopathy or herbal medicine, then Shiatsu can perhaps help prevent its recurrence. The basic treatment principle will be to strengthen all the Organs in the body connected with eliminating waste products; namely the Kidney, Bladder, Large Intestine and Lungs. Strengthening the Kidney and Bladder will improve detoxification of the blood via the excretion of urine. Working on the Large Intestine will help by facilitating bowel movements. The net result will be to take the strain off the skin; itself an organ of elimination. Therefore, Channels for special attention would be the Kidney and Large Intestine Channels, and also the Lung Channel, because the Lungs supply Ki and moisture to the skin.

PSYCHOSIS

Psychosis differs from neurosis insofar as the individual loses contact with reality. Psychosis is commonly referred to as 'madness'. Schizophrenia and manic depressive illness are two examples of psychotic behaviour. Shiatsu could have a role similar to that described for neurosis (see page 141), but the result would probably be minimal. On the other hand, if everybody gave each other basic 'grassroots' Shiatsu, as a process of normal social interaction, psychosis and other psychological disorders would doubtless be less prevalent.

RESPIRATORY DISORDERS

Shiatsu can do a lot for most respiratory disorders, of which there are many. Most respiratory disorders can be approached with similar treatment principles as those described for Asthma (page 104) and Bronchitis (page 107).

RHEUMATOID ARTHRITIS

See Arthritis, page 103.

RUNNING INJURIES

Running injuries are common, but most could be prevented if the balance of the posture was finely tuned. Shiatsu and Sotai corrective exercises do exactly that, amongst other things. Muscle and ligament injuries are common running injuries. Their specific relationship to Shiatsu treatment is described under Muscle Strain (page 140) and Ligament Sprain (page 134).

SACROILIAC STRAIN

This is where the ligaments providing the connection between the sacrum and the pelvis become sprained. Osteopathic manipulation can help in some cases. However, the fine balancing of the pelvis possible through Sotai corrective exercises is one of the very best treatments for this. Shiatsu to the Kidney, Bladder, Small Intestine and Liver Channels is also of considerable benefit. This is because the Bladder Channel, supported by the Kidney Channel extension, supplies Ki to the sacroiliac area. Resultant tension in the buttock muscles can be released by stretching and dispersing the Small Intestine Channel extension in the legs. The Liver Channel is good to treat because it controls the nourishment of ligaments.

SCHIZOPHRENIA

See Psychosis, page 149.

SCIATICA

Sciatica is the term given to pain that radiates along the sciatic nerve. The pain affects the buttocks and back of the thighs and sometimes also the leg and foot. It may also cause numbness, pins and needles and/or weakness in those areas. The most common cause is prolapse of an intervertebral disc (slipped disc) in the lumbar region, causing pressure on the sciatic nerve. It can also be caused by a tumour, abscess, sciatic nerve inflammation, or an awkward sitting posture.

Careful Shiatsu techniques to decompress and lengthen the lumbar vertebrae may be effective. These involve gentle stretching and relaxing of the lumbar musculature, deep soft tissue manipulation through the belly, rebalancing of the Bladder and

Kidney Channels and the Large Intestine and Small Intestine Channel extensions (all of which lie in close proximity to the sciatic nerve pathway). Sotai corrective exercises are excellent. Many cases respond well to osteopathy or chiropractic. If the cause is not clear, it is important to be medically examined to highlight any possible non-structural causes such as an abscess or a tumour.

SCOLIOSIS

Scoliosis is the term used for a sideways distortion of the thoracic vertebrae. Severe cases show as an expanded area on one side of the upper back. Scoliosis may be 'fixed', meaning that an irreversible bone deformity is present, or it may be 'non-fixed', meaning that it results from a pelvis which is tilted out of line. Pelvic misalignment can usually be helped by Sotai corrective exercises, Shiatsu, osteopathy or chiropractic. Extensive Shiatsu to the Gall Bladder Channel can rebalance the right and left sides of the body, thus helping to re-align the pelvis.

SHOCK

The body reacts to severe physical or emotional trauma by going into shock. Shock is essentially a sudden and extreme reduction in the flow of blood to the tissues. This causes the person to become cold, clammy and pale, with sweating, nausea and sometimes vomiting. If it occurs following an injury, medical assistance should be called immediately. For mild cases of shock, Shiatsu can help by increasing the warming (more Yang) levels of Ki in the body. This can be achieved by tonifying the Kidney Channel, especially working on the first point of the Kidney Channel on the sole of the foot. Other specific points and techniques to increase the blood circulation would be used.

In some cases, moxibustion (see page 162) would be applied to specific points in order to generate heat quickly.

Experience reveals that in the case of emotional shock, the Small Intestine Channel becomes very depleted. Consequently, tonification of the Small Intestine Channel is very helpful. The Heart and Heart Protector Channels might also require some attention.

Note that shock also responds very well to homoeopathy and Bach flower remedies.

SHOULDER STIFFNESS

Shoulder stiffness may be the symptom of an injury or of a frozen shoulder (see page 122); or it may occur for no obvious reason. Because the Channels of Ki flow all around and through this most mobile of joints, any distortion in the Channels elsewhere in the body will cause a jamming-up of Ki in the shoulder. In other words, any postural or organic dysfunction in the body can very easily result in shoulder stiffness. Imbalances in the Large Intestine and Small Intestine Channels will almost always give some degree of shoulder pain. A full body Shiatsu to deal with underlying imbalances, preceded by and followed by a comprehensive routine of techniques to the shoulder, will invariably help. For undiagnosed shoulder stiffness, Shiatsu is by far the most appropriate option to take. However, acupuncture and physiotherapy are usually effective also.

SINUSITIS

Treatment as for Nasal Congestion (see page 140).

SLIPPED DISC

See Sciatica, page 150.

SORE THROAT

A sore throat often accompanies colds or flu. It may also be due to a local bacterial infection in the throat. In Oriental Medicine, it represents Heat in the Lungs and upper airways. The Shiatsu therapist will give vigorous dispersing techniques to the Lung and Large Intestine Channels in the arms, particularly focusing upon the hands. This will cool the Lungs and throat and help clear excess Heat from the body. Note that herbal medicine is the best treatment for sore throats.

SPASTIC PARALYSIS

Spastic paralysis is the inability to move a part of the body because of extreme tension and rigidity in the muscle. It may be caused by a stroke (see Hemiplegia, page 125) or any injury or disease of the brain and spinal cord. Shiatsu, like Physiotherapy, is able to reduce spasticity by gently coaxing the affected muscles to relax. General Shiatsu, when done in a calming, focused way, can relieve spasticity dramatically. However, it needs to be repeated frequently to prevent contractures (permanent muscle shortening resulting from chronic, unrelieved, spastic muscle contraction).

SPORTS INJURIES

Sports injuries are effectively dealt with by physiotherapists and osteopaths. Many sports injuries involve muscle strain and ligament sprain. These are dealt with on pages 140 and 134 respectively.

SPRAIN

See Ligament Sprain, page 134.

STAMMERING

Stammering, also called stuttering, usually starts in very early childhood, often persisting into adulthood. However, it can start in adulthood if the Ki within the Heart and Heart Protector Channels becomes congested or overactive (the Heart controls the tongue and therefore affects speech). This may arise from severe anxiety. Calming of the Heart and Heart Protector Channels will help. Shiatsu cannot easily help stammering which is rooted in early childhood. Speech therapists are the obvious therapists for this situation.

STRESS

Most of us are subject to stress factors which inhibit the realization of maximum health in the way nature intended. This is not entirely our fault as individuals, for even if we eat, work, sleep and play in the right way, we are still subject to external stresses and pollutants which undermine our natural self-healing ability. Clearly, we do not live in a garden of Eden where everything is untainted, or where everyone goes out of their way to make us happy. Stress and tension are easy to come by and most of us have experienced enough stress to make a detailed description of its many effects superfluous. Suffice it to remind ourselves that tiredness, frustration, irritability and increased susceptibility to disease go hand in hand with excessive stress.

Stress in itself is not problematic. It sharpens our reflexes and drives us on to higher goals. It is excessive relentless stress which wears down our ability to bounce straight back to health.

One of the things that exacerbates the effects of stress is lack of positive support from other human beings. The well-worn saying 'a problem shared is a problem halved' is certainly true. Shiatsu offers more than specific pressure point treatment and techniques; it offers communication and support through touch.

Touch from another human being, given with empathy and rapport, is in itself de-stressing. It activates the parasympathetic nervous system which is responsible for calming us down. Stressful situations activate the sympathetic nervous system which stimulates the flow of adrenalin and generally prepares us for challenge. Unrelenting stressful situations which are not balanced by proper relaxation result in the body being stuck in the sympathetic 'keyed up' state. This results in muscular tension, anxiety, insomnia and eventually exhaustion of the adrenal glands.

Consequently, the way in which Shiatsu can help alleviate the effects of stress is to apply non-invasive touch from an attitude of sensitivity and compassion, encouraging relaxation and 'letting go', as opposed to intrusive touch which instantly causes the recipient to tense up even more and withdraw.

The treatment principles described for anxiety (see page 100) apply equally to stress.

STROKE

See Hemiplegia, page 125.

TENNIS ELBOW

Tennis elbow is pain on the outside of the elbow resulting from inflammation of the tendon which attaches there. It is caused by overuse of the elbow joint during certain activities such as tennis, gardening and lifting heavy objects. A similar condition called golfer's elbow results from inflammation of the tendon attached to the inside of the elbow. Complete rest of the forearm muscles by applying a special splint is usually the best treatment. Shiatsu can help relieve the pain by applying pressure to all the pressure points around the elbow which are not tender. For tennis elbow, Shiatsu technique to the Large Intestine Channel either side of the elbow in the forearm and upper arm can help. For golfer's elbow, similar techniques to the Heart and Small Intestine Channels can help.

TENSION

Psychological tension is the feeling of being unpleasantly keyed up because of mental strain, bottled-up emotions and anxiety. Physical tension usually accompanies psychological tension and results in headaches and muscular stiffness with pain. The stiffness and pain focus particularly in the upper back and shoulders. On a purely symptomatic level of immediate relief, dispersing style Shiatsu to the areas concerned works wonders. Cross fibre stretching, as described under muscle stiffness (page 138) is an effective technique for the back. To deal with the underlying anxiety and stress see Anxiety (page 100) and Stress (page 154). Meditation, Yoga and Qi Gong are all excellent for reducing tension.

THROMBOSIS

If a doctor tells you that you have a thrombosis, it means that you have a blood clot within a blood vessel. A common example is deep vein thrombosis, which is a clot within the deep-lying veins of the legs. The doctor may treat this with anti-coagulant drugs. **Do not seek Shiatsu treatment** if you suspect or know you have a thrombus (thrombosis). The techniques of Shiatsu may cause part of the thrombus to break loose and lodge somewhere else in the circulatory system. If it lodges in the brain, a stroke may result. If it lodges in the heart, it may cause a heart attack.

TINNITUS

Tinnitus is ringing, hissing, buzzing or whistling sounds in the ears, which are heard in the absence of those sounds in the environment. It can occur as a symptom of many ear disorders. It may also be present for no apparent reason.

Oriental Medicine recognizes Kidney imbalance to be one cause of tinnitus. However, tinnitus in general is very difficult to treat successfully. Chinese herbs and acupuncture are sometimes successful. Shiatsu may help via tonification of the Kidney and Bladder Channels, plus rebalancing of the Gall Bladder, Triple Heater and Governing Vessel Channels in the head.

TOOTHACHE

A toothache must have an underlying cause, which should be ascertained and treated by a dentist. However, Shiatsu can be of great help in easing the pain until such time as the dentist can see you. Dispersing techniques applied to the armpit, upper chest, upper arm and shoulder area are effective. These techniques you can apply to yourself.

Upper toothache – Firmly squeeze the deltoid muscle, located on the cap of the shoulder.

Lower toothache – Firmly squeeze the pectoralis major muscle, located close to the front of the armpit.

For upper toothache, the Shiatsu therapist would also apply strong pressure along the Heart and Small Intestine Channels on the outside of the arm. For lower toothache, strong pressure to the Lung and Large Intestine Channels in the hand may help.

Gum pain can be helped by applying firm pressure to the Heart Protector Channel along the centre line of the inner arm.

TOXAEMIA

Toxaemia is the presence of poisons in the blood. Herbal medicine has a wide variety of plants and extracts excellent for cleansing the blood, and for strengthening and activating the body's eliminating systems. Unless the eliminatory systems, such as the Kidneys and Large Intestine, are functioning well, it is difficult to get the poisons out of the body.

Shiatsu can strengthen and stimulate the Kidneys and Large Intestine, thus improving elimination. Additional Shiatsu to the Liver, Gall Bladder and Stomach Channels will also help.

TRAVEL SICKNESS

This can be alleviated by applying firm pressure into a point called Heart Protector 6 or 'inner gate'. This point lies in the middle of the lower inner forearm, two thumb widths above the wrist crease. Keep the pressure on until the symptoms of nausea retreat. Chewing a little piece of ginger root or drinking some peppermint tea usually helps.

VARICOSE VEINS

Varicose veins are swollen, twisted superficial veins, most commonly present in the legs. They can also occur in the anus, where they are called haemorrhoids or piles. Varicose veins result from defective valves in the vein wall, which cause pooling of blood and consequent swelling in the veins. Obesity, hormonal changes and pressure on the pelvis during pregnancy can all contribute to their development. However, Oriental Medicine recognizes that weakness of the Ki associated with the Heart and Spleen may encourage their development. Therefore, Shiatsu given to the Heart Channel and

Spleen Channel to strengthen and 'tighten' the veins, can help
prevent them.

VERTIGO

Vertigo is disorientation due to the illusion that one's surroundings are spinning. It results from a disturbance of the balance mechanisms in the ear. Unless it is a symptom of some physical disorder, it is usually associated with fear of heights.

Vertigo is essentially a state of being extremely ungrounded. Highly focused and supportive Shiatsu to the belly and feet will dramatically increase the recipient's sense of grounding and stability, both physically and mentally. Working on the Stomach and Spleen Channels in the legs will consolidate this, because these are the Channels of the Earth Element, and therefore most associated with being grounded. In addition, rebalancing of the Gall Bladder Channel to aid balance, plus tonification of the Kidney Channel to help the ears and reduce phobia, can be very effective.

WHIPLASH INJURIES

This is injury to the ligaments, muscles and joints of the neck resulting from car collisions or other accidents involving sudden acceleration or deceleration.

The severity of the injury determines the treatment. Where the spinal cord is at risk, medical attention is required. Less severe cases can be treated by osteopaths or chiropractors. Mild cases can be helped by Sotai corrective exercises and Shiatsu. The Small Intestine and Triple Heater Channels are often distorted following a whiplash. Therefore, the Shiatsu therapist is likely to spend some time rebalancing them. Shiatsu to the lower back, hips and legs will also be given, because neck alignment largely depends upon correct lower body alignment.

ADJUNCTS TO SHIATSU THEORY AND PRACTICE

REACTIONS TO TREATMENT AND THE LAWS OF CURE

I t is possible, although uncommon, to feel temporary discomforts or mild disorientation during or after receiving
Shiatsu. These reactions usually only happen when the
body contains a lot of accumulated toxins which begin to be
expelled as a result of the treatment. Such reactions need not
cause undue concern. They are, in fact, an indication that an
internal cleansing of the body is taking place. This is therefore a
beneficial process, but if it should happen to you, do not hesi-
tate to notify your Shiatsu therapist. He or she will be able to
reassure you, and give relevant advice. These reactions rarely
occur more than once, but if they do, they will always be less
severe with subsequent treatments.

There is a process called the 'Laws of Cure' which clarifies the
meaning of reactions to treatment. The Laws of Cure were for-
mulated by Constantin Hering, a famous homoeopath who
observed certain phenomena when sick patients became cured.
His observations are as applicable to Oriental Medicine as they
are to homoeopathy. Hering's Laws of Cure state that as someone is cured, the following may occur:

- Symptoms move from within to without.
  This means that if someone has a serious heart problem, they may experience bowel or skin problems during the process of cure.

- Cure takes place from above to below.
  As healing takes place, symptoms usually leave as if they were 'dripping off' the body. For example, a pain in the head will leave first, followed by a pain in the back, with a pain or rash in the hands or feet to be the last to go. Symptoms can also migrate downwards so that a headache can *become* a backache, which becomes a rash on the foot.

- Previous symptoms will be experienced in reverse chronological order.
  Symptoms that were previously suppressed often resurface during the process of cure and usually do so in reverse order from their original sequence. For example, asthma often occurs in people who once suffered from eczema which was apparently cured (but really only suppressed) by steroid-based lotions. The eczema, having merely been driven deeper into the body, may re-emerge after the asthma has been successfully treated. Symptoms re-experienced are usually much less severe than they were first time around. In fact they can reappear simply as a dream. Thus, some time after treatment, the asthma sufferer may dream of having eczema.

It is impossible to predict how severe Law of Cure reactions will be, or whether they will appear at all. However, their occurrence is a positive indication of recovery. I believe it is important for patients to understand this law because those who are unaware of it may cease treatment believing they are getting worse.

Physical reactions are most likely to occur after treatment. However, it is possible to have an emotional reaction during a

PRINCIPLES OF SHIATSU

treatment. This is because the recipient may open up to reveal a hidden and vulnerable part of themselves, in order to get some support in strengthening a weakness, or discharging a problem which has been troubling the psyche. However, this is only likely to happen after a great deal of trust and rapport has accumulated between therapist and patient, or if the therapist is particularly adept at dealing with such situations. It will not happen with the inexperienced practitioner.

MOXIBUSTION

Moxibustion is a method used by many Shiatsu therapists and acupuncturists for increasing warmth (Yang) in the body, thereby dispelling coldness and Ki stagnation. It involves the burning of a herb, similar to mugwort, called *Artemisia vulgaris* or 'moxa'. Moxa can be applied in three ways:

a. A small amount is burnt directly upon the skin, over a Tsubo, and removed when the heat is felt, but before the skin is burnt.
b. It is applied as above, but with a bed of ginger or salt between the moxa and the skin. This method eliminates the risk of burning the skin.
c. A 'moxa stick' is held over a Tsubo, without touching the skin.

Most Shiatsu therapists who use moxibustion favour the 'moxa stick' method. One advantage of this is that the stick can be passed slowly along a Channel pathway, or across the belly of a muscle. This gives a more general tonifying effect upon the Ki flow within Channels, and upon blood circulation.

Because moxibustion is used for warming, it will only be given to people who have symptoms of Cold. Generally, it is not useful for those who have symptoms of Heat.

Britain and the rest of North-west Europe is a cold, damp region in comparison to the Mediterranean and most other areas. As such, most of us could use a little warming up in Winter. Consequently, moxibustion is a very applicable form of treatment for use in this part of the world.

Several Tsubos have contraindications to the use of moxa. Certain medical disorders also negate its use. Therefore, do not be tempted to buy a moxa stick and use it randomly upon yourself or others. Sometimes the therapist will give you one to use at home. If this happens, only use it on those areas of the body suggested to you.

SOTAI

Sotai is a System of exercises which rebalance postural distortions. Its basic technique is to discover which movements in the body are stiff and painful, and then to work away from the stiffness and pain. For example, pain on the left side of the neck on turning your head to the left would be treated by the therapist applying a light resistance to the head as it is turned to the right. This is repeated two or three times. Consequently, the stiffness and pain is reduced and it becomes easier to turn the head to the left.

This approach contrasts with the common assumption that exercising into the stiff areas of the body will create more movement.

CASE HISTORIES AND OTHER APPLICATIONS

THE STORY OF MR G

Patient G had been receiving Shiatsu once a week for nine months to boost his vitality, and thus enable him to cope better with the pressures of his demanding job as a physician. This was quite successful, until he unexpectedly began to deteriorate in health.

Mr G's original presentation was of a lack of vitality, with constant Kyo (lack of Ki) within his Kidney Channel. His Ki was not very strong or consistent anywhere. In addition he had a definite pallor to his complexion, weakness in his legs and loose stools. Emotionally he was rather reserved and self-conscious.

This person was a particularly clear archetype of someone with lack of strength in the Kidneys. The cause of this weakness was largely both hereditary and occupational insofar as he was a person of frail constitution locked in a non-physical yet mentally exhausting job. Nothing about his diet could be isolated as an aggravating factor.

My treatment aims were to tonify his Kidneys and to help him discover a little more self-assurance. My main approach was to concentrate on nurturing the core of his energy and strength by way of deep tonification of the belly and the

Bladder Channel in the lower back. I encouraged him throughout to focus on any feelings of 'connection' and warmth in his belly and to visualize this as a strong 'recharging' of his batteries. In addition I applied moxa to some Tsubos in the lower back, and then focused on tonifying the Kidney Channel in the chest, for the purpose of strengthening confidence. After six treatments over three weeks he had a significant increase in vitality which he sustained for the following six months, receiving Shiatsu thereafter, once each week.

In October 1986, G began to experience some mild asthma attacks which coincided with an increase in responsibility at work and the return of his Kidney weakness, plus a full (Jitsu) quality to his Lung Channel. He had experienced asthma only once before, as a young teenager.

I treated him in much the same way as before, but included a well-tried technique called 'tonifying the two Sea of Ki points', (see Fig 51 on page 107) in an attempt to help the Kidneys pull the Ki down from the Lung. This involves holding light, focused touch over Tsubos Directing Vessel 6 and 17, while encouraging the recipient to relate to a sense of 'connection' between the two. This was supported by some other techniques which have a similar effect. I gave him some appropriate herbs and he was fine for a while.

Six weeks later G exhibited a Spleen uncharacteristically more Kyo than his Kidneys. I tonified Kyo wherever I found it and focused my Ki very strongly on his belly. Nothing positive happened between treatments so the following week I gave a particularly supportive and nurturing Shiatsu to boost the strength of the Earth Element within him. The next treatment saw him feeling very cold and well under par, so I applied moxa to the various appropriate Tsubos. I told him to keep warm, eat warm foods, and *think* warm. He felt slightly better for three weeks, then got flu symptoms lasting for five weeks, during which time I did not treat him. When I was satisfied his flu had completely gone I gave him a herbal formula, as I was concerned about the strength of his immune system. He felt better, although still weak, for a month.

When I saw G at the end of March 1987, he looked emaciated and was losing a lot of hair; not as in male pattern baldness syndrome, but in clumps. I told him that I could not fathom why his general health was deteriorating, and asked when he had last received a medical check-up. This was really a hint to get him to see a doctor. He said he had seen a doctor two months ago, who confirmed he had full blown AIDS. It seems G had suspected this for several months, but had declined to tell me.

G expressed his concern that I might deter from giving him Shiatsu given the nature of his condition. However, I reassured him that I was more than willing to proceed. He realized, as I did, that he could not expect a cure from Shiatsu, but felt it was helpful on other levels. G was very 'matter-of-fact' in the way he talked about things of grave consequence to himself, but clearly this situation required the maximum sensitivity and tact on my part. He greatly appreciated the physical contact afforded by Shiatsu and respected my deliberate 'you're in no way different from anybody else' approach.

From then on I applied everything I could think of to help nurture the remnants of G's immune system, and suggested other therapists with other skills (in particular a Chinese herbalist and homoeopath). Fortunately he had daily access to people (counsellors and psychotherapists) whom I knew would give him exceptional psychological and emotional support. Despite this his physical condition progressively deteriorated until he ended up with a heart pacemaker and all sorts of tubes plugged into his lungs. I really thought he was reaching his final days. He then told me that the only thing which made him feel human and in any way positive was the Shiatsu sessions. I asked him if he was ready or prepared to 'go' yet. He said 'no'.

At G's request I began to treat him three to five times per week. I soon found the most effective Shiatsu treatment was to warm and tonify the belly area for 10 to 15 minutes, then to tonify the completely Kyo Triple Heater Channel in the thighs for up to 45 minutes. It is the Triple Heater which directs the Ki from the reservoir of Ki in the belly to every Organ and Channel of the body, thereby warming and protecting them. Also, by extending this Ki to the body's periphery, the Triple Heater facilitates the Defensive Ki in protecting the body. Remarkably, after six weeks G had got rid of all the paraphernalia inserted into his body. Thereafter I did virtually the same treatment as just described regularly twice per week.

G seemed to maintain a status quo for almost a year until one day he was admitted to hospital quite suddenly, and fitted with a full complement of tubes and and gadgets. I visited him and asked him: 'Are you throwing in the towel, G?' (though not quite that bluntly), and he said 'not yet'. He also asked me if I would come and give him Shiatsu. I said I would, but must confess I felt very nervous doing it in a hospital ward. Fortunately he got himself into a single 'hospice' room. Being a doctor himself, he convinced the hospital staff to accept anything I might do to him.

By the next time I saw G, he had developed a mixture of very severe symptoms. These symptoms may have been aggravated by the powerful medication he was on at the time. I knew of certain Chinese herbs which would be relevant, but felt he needed someone a bit more experienced with herbs to prescribe them. I arranged that immediately. Meanwhile I used moxa on some relevant Tsubos, followed by sustained pressure on all Kyo areas of the Kidney and Spleen Channels that I could get at.

G had perked up a lot when I saw him next, and seemed relatively OK for about a month. Then one day I came to give one of his housemates a Shiatsu, and she informed me that G had passed away overnight. She said: 'He asked me to tell you he feels OK about going, and said the Shiatsu helped to make it so'.

G was a very sensitive and philosophical individual, who responded well to the subtle aspects of support and connection within a Shiatsu session. I consider the Shiatsu to have been successful on several levels, although in the end he died. However, I sincerely believe he *was* 'OK' about that in the end; perhaps even in the beginning.

A STORY WITH A HAPPY ENDING – A CHANGE OF RHYTHM

Jackie Keirs is a dancer and choreographer, and author of *A Change of Rhythm*, a book describing her recovery from a serious road accident. She has written about dance in education and recently made a video on the same subject. She is founder/ director of the Oxford Dance Theatre. This is Jackie's story in her own words.

'In 1978 I was involved in a traffic accident. An articulated lorry jack-knifed and landed on top of my car, a Mini, as I was driving between two schools after a CSE dance assessment. Fortunately, the accident took place very near Stoke Mandeville Hospital and, having been cut out of the car, I was taken there by ambulance and operated on immediately. I had sustained a serious head injury which was followed by three weeks of concussion, paralysis, loss of speech and memory, double vision, plus complete physical, mental and emotional turmoil.

'However, I seemed to make a very quick recovery. I was back at school teaching full-time in less than six months. But this recovery proved illusory. Within two years I began to have abnormal feelings of tension, particularly in my head, and by the time I left the school to become freelance in 1980 this discomfort had become pain, later diagnosed by the Abingdon Pain Relief Clinic as a very rare but recognized syndrome, thalamic pain. Since that time, having written a book about it and appeared on television, I have got to know of four other people in England who have been diagnosed as having the same syndrome. I have no idea how many more there may be.

'I was given a variety of drug treatments, none of which worked for any length of time. I had ganglion block injections in the neck, to stop the nerve impulses to the brain. At least I believe this was the purpose; it was never properly explained to me. Finally, a decision was made to settle with the drug Anxon as being more tolerable than any other, enabling me partially to regulate the pain. I stayed on that drug for about seven years. All the time I was trying alternatives: acupuncture, homoeopathy, massage, radionics, touch for health; becoming increasingly desperate, but nothing was able effectively to reverse the pain.

'Anxon had been privatized in 1985, making it impossible to obtain on prescription, and then Beechams started producing it in smaller quantities. I wrote asking for reassurance that they would continue making it, only to be told that they would "soon discontinue the product altogether". They advised me to try one of the many "products very similar to Anxon" prescribable by my own GP. When I went to the chemist in August last year to collect my next dose I found that the drugs had been withdrawn overnight. They were no longer financially viable.

'The effects of coming off anxiety relievers like these can be as bad as those caused by coming off hard narcotics, as I was soon to learn to my cost. I was on the relatively "small dose" of one pill a day, so I dread to think how anyone who had been on a higher dose spent last summer! I had to cope with the withdrawal symptoms of coming off Anxon together with the side effects of

Tegratol, a drug which I had tried before but which was now being given to me in increasingly large doses.

'I had suffered the pain for ten years and learned to live with it. I had it every day, in my head, face, arm, hand, and worst of all, eyes, from about midday onwards. It was infinitely wearying and meant that I had to rest every afternoon just to make the day shorter and to enable me to do what helped me more than anything to survive the pain – dance. Although I only occasionally performed, dance in all its aspects – teaching, choreography and recently, directing – was definitely the focal point of my life. It was a totally absorbing way of channelling the energy left me by the pain, the only worthwhile distraction I could find, since everything else which involved contact with people only served to make the pain more acute. Above all it was the most powerful way of expressing my pain. I had to communicate it somehow, and if it bored people to listen to me prattling on about it, then I would dance.

'I felt very strongly that there had to be some point to the suffering, that it should find an outlet for expression, and that I was lucky, in a rather perverse way, to have at my fingertips the means to express it artistically. By dancing I was able to experience the pain more deeply, to investigate it, to use it, to rise above it, to take it beyond itself and articulate it powerfully for others. It was a dance about my pain that Central Television featured in their documentary about me, broadcast as one of the Link programmes in 1986. In its physicality, dance is close to pain; prose is inadequate. I did once spontaneously describe it, to the then head of the Pain Relief Clinic at Abingdon, as "scything, searing, corroding, corrupting". He told me to stop being poetic.

'For eight years then, there had been two real obsessions in my life: dance and pain. It was a fantastic challenge just to get through a day, and every day I would be testing my will power to see if I was equal to the task. Two things prevented me from committing suicide: I was not brave enough and had no wish to hurt my mother. I had no fear of death itself. In fact I would have preferred it.

'So, somehow or other, I coped. Then my drugs were taken off the market. It was as if the ground had been taken from under my feet and I was gradually reduced to a cipher of myself. The pain became daily more acute, I wept continually, my double vision and dizziness grew infinitely worse. The one effect of which the GP had warned me, that I might get a "dry mouth", was nowhere amongst this maelstrom of sensations. I was unable to drive and could barely walk into town. Moreover, sleep was impossible, although I wrapped myself in hot scarves to disguise the pain, wore ear plugs to cut out the noise and regularly took four sleeping pills a night. I just about managed to keep teaching, but only for an hour or two a day. Any semblance of normal life, let alone dancing and directing, became inconceivable. Why, I wonder, are drug companies not obliged by law to list for the consumer the potential side-effects of their products?

'Finally I gave up. I said to a friend, "I can't go on"; it was the first time in ten years that I had been able to bring myself to articulate the thought in words. He took me to the doctor's surgery but neither of the two doctors conversant with my case was there. The doctor who was did not want to take any decisions, and had no advice to offer. I went straight to another friend, yet another shoulder to cry on, to ask for suggestions how I might improve my situation. She had heard of a therapy that I had not tried yet. A friend had apparently said good things about it. This was Shiatsu.

'By this stage, even to leave my house felt beyond me, so Sally,* the Shiatsu therapist, came to me. Her first reactions were set out in a letter to my doctor:

"I could see as soon as I met her that Jackie was indeed on

*Sally is the course director of the European Shiatsu School's Oxford branch.

PRINCIPLES OF SHIATSU

the point of mental collapse and only sheer determination was keeping her going. Her body looked frail, as if a puff of wind could blow it away."

'She laid me on a mattress on the floor and without saying or asking anything, gave me a very quiet, healing treatment. Kneeling beside me she held me very gently. My memory is of an invigorating human warmth. Paradoxically, I grew very cold and had to be wrapped in blankets. Afterwards, I felt a little more buoyant and arranged another treatment a few days later.

'It was that evening I began to feel different. I drove a short way to see a friend, and instead of my hands falling off the wheel, as they had been doing, I felt stronger and more relaxed, and had no pain in my head.

'Since then I have not looked back. I have been able to come off my drugs in less than two months, and am now able to glimpse a life relatively free of pain. At the beginning I was having treatments three or four times a week, as I felt unable to live without them, but gradually I have become stronger, and can now survive on only one. I am not without uncomfortable sensations, but they no longer engulf me in the way the pain used to. For the first time in several years my eyes are clear, I can touch and taste, and my body is full of wonderful sensations. After years of dryness, my mouth is full of bubbles. My hair feels thick, soft and silky, my hands like pearls.'

NOTE:

Shiatsu is not always *that* successful every time, but it is encouraging to know that it can initiate such powerful and positive changes in people.

Jackie received the *'Here's Health* Achiever of the Year Award' of 1991, for her success in overcoming her problems.

SHIATSU FOR BABIES AND YOUNG CHILDREN

In Japan, basic Shiatsu is practised within the family as part of daily life. We in the west could be of great benefit to our children if we did likewise. Short foundation courses in basic Shiatsu techniques are available to every interested parent nationwide through the European Shiatsu School and other organizations (see resources section at the end of this book).

Beyond any application Shiatsu may have in healing, it is of general benefit to children because it develops greater bonding between the child and the parent. In addition, it enables the parent greater opportunity to notice any physical abnormalities or structural misalignments. If any physical anomalies are discovered, the parent can seek the relevant professional help to correct the problem. It is well worth discovering such anomalies sooner rather than later. Finally, Shiatsu is worth giving to children just because they find it such fun to receive.

Shiatsu to babies under 18 months old involves a light stroking action along their Channels, rather than the use of pressure. For Children between 18 months and four years, it is still better to avoid pressure in favour of rocking and rubbing techniques. Beyond four years of age, most Shiatsu techniques can be used. However, because a child's attention span is short, they respond better to active dispersing-style techniques rather than static tonification techniques. Children are rarely deficiency in Ki anyway, so they do not usually require tonification.

Difficult, hard-to-handle children can benefit immensely from Shiatsu, provided you can coax them into receiving it in the first place. After succeeding in getting them to receive it once, you should be able to persuade them fairly easily thereafter. Children with cerebral palsy derive particularly great benefit from Shiatsu (see page 110).

SHIATSU FOR THE ELDERLY

People become less flexible and more frail as they get older, and so require Shiatsu which is more gentle. The positions for receiving Shiatsu may need to be modified to maintain comfort, and the room will need to be extra warm. Many techniques can be done in a chair, so there is no excuse for any elderly or infirm person to miss out on this incredibly supportive bodywork. Remember, being old does not mean being devoid of the need for physical contact.

SHIATSU AS A PREVENTATIVE THERAPY

Earlier in this book we have seen how Shiatsu can be of help in the treatment of various disorders. In general, most people tend to wait until ill-health develops before seeking help to combat their disorder. However, there is a growing trend towards health consciousness whereby many people are taking positive steps to reduce the likelihood of becoming ill. This health consciousness not only reflects concern for the physical body, for example, by eating more sensibly and exercising, but for the mind also.

Shiatsu can be of considerable benefit in helping us all stay healthy or become healthier, because it corrects distortions in the energies supplying both body and mind. As such, regular Shiatsu treatment will detect and deal with our energetic distortions before they create troublesome symptoms. The overall relaxing effect of Shiatsu is also of great benefit in preventing imbalances arising.

The role of Shiatsu as a preventative therapy is rather akin to 'fine tuning' a musical instrument. When a musical instrument is out of tune, musical disharmony results. Musical disharmony not only affects the poor state of balance within the instrument, but it affects the sense of harmony within all who are listening. Perhaps therefore, the harmony within individuals is partially dependent on the harmony within surrounding individuals. If as many people as possible could stay firmly 'tuned' and in balance, maybe the orchestra of humanity would play a more harmonious tune.

Shiatsu is therefore not only about personal health, but potentially about social health as well. After all, the first step towards understanding each other is to make contact with each other. Surely, the most profound form of contact is through aware and supportive touch.

So, how often should we receive Shiatsu? It would be nice to receive it every day. However, most of us could only afford the time and expense to have one or two sessions per week. Having a Shiatsu once per month is a good way to stop your energies wandering too far out of tune. Irrespective of how often you think you might like to receive Shiatsu, a course of three or four sessions is recommended to enable you to feel its full potential. If you are ill or injured, then a few more treatments may be required. The best thing to do is to learn the basics together with a friend, and swap 'grassroots' Shiatsu. That way you can receive it for its relaxing benefits more often, and at more flexible times. You will also discover the joy and benefits of giving Shiatsu as well as receiving it. About fifty hours of tuition (four weekends) would give you enough skill to relax and de-stress a friend, although it takes a minimum of three years to become a proficient practitioner with developed diagnostic skills.

RESOURCES

WHERE TO RECEIVE TUITION OR TREATMENTS

Shiatsu tuition is very widely available throughout Britain and Europe. Within Britain all legitimate Schools of Shiatsu are affiliated to the Shiatsu Society, which was founded in 1981 as an independent representative body for everyone involved in Shiatsu. Its officers are elected from the membership, which is open to anyone with a keen interest in Shiatsu. The society operates an independent assessment panel governing entry onto the Practitioner register. All registered Practitioners use the initials MRSS (Member of The Register of the Shiatsu Society).

The more established Shiatsu Schools are:

The European Shiatsu School – London and branch schools networked throughout major cities in Britain and Europe. Details of all ESS schools can be obtained from ESS Central Administration, Highbanks, Lockeridge, Marlborough, Wilts SN8 4EQ.

Bristol School of Shiatsu and Oriental Medicine – Bristol (affiliated to the European Shiatsu School)

British School of Shiatsu – Do – London

The Devon School of Shiatsu – Totnes

The East Anglia School of Shiatsu – Ipswich

The Glasgow School of Shiatsu – Glasgow

Healing Shiatsu Education Centre – Hereford

Ki Kai Shiatsu Centre – London

The Shiatsu College – London

Further details and addresses of all these Shiatsu Schools, plus a complete register of qualified Shiatsu practitioners, can be obtained from the Shiatsu Society Secretary, 14 Oakdene Rd, Redhill, Surrey RH1 6BT.

RECOMMENDED BOOKS

By the same author:
Shiatsu: The Complete Guide (Thorsons)
Acupressure for Common Ailments (Gaia Books)

Other titles:
The Foundations of Chinese Medicine, Giovanni Maciocia
   (Churchill Livingstone)
Zen Shiatsu, Shizuto Masunaga (Japan Publications)
The Book of Shiatsu, Paul Lundberg (Gaia Books)
Shiatsu Workbook: A Beginner's Guide, Nigel Dawes (Piatkus)
A Beginner's Guide to Shiatsu, Jane Downer (Hodder and
   Stoughton)
The Theory & Practice of Shiatsu, Carola Beresford-Cook
   (Churchill Livingstone)

INDEX

acupuncture 35, 69, 95
   passim
addiction 94–5
AIDS 95–6, 128
   case history 164–8
aims of Shiatsu 37
Alexander technique 99, 103, 106,
   135
allergies 96
anaemia 96–7
anger 67
angina pectoris 97–8
ankylosing spondylitis 99
anorexia nervosa 100
anxiety 100–102
appendectomy 102
aromatherapy 105, 108, 139
arteriosclerosis 103
arthritis 103–4
asking 73–4
assessment, Shiatsu health 72–6
asthma 104–5
atherosclerosis 98, 103

babies and Shiatsu 173
Bach Flower Remedies 114, 128,
   141, 144, 152
back pain 105–6
balance, importance of 33, 83,
   141

Bell's palsy 119
benefits of Shiatsu 87–92
Bladder, function of 48–9
bleeding, internal 89
Blood 8
   and Heart 41, 53–4
   and Internal Organs 41
   and Liver 41
   and Spleen 41, 50–52
blood clots 89
blood pressure
   high 127
   low 135
Body Fluids 8
   and Heart 43
   and Internal Organs 42–3
   and Kidneys 42
   and Lungs 42
   and Spleen 42
body parts to avoid 89–90
bonding 173
breath, steadiness of 80, 144
bronchitis 107
bruising 90, 108
bulimia 108
burns 90, 108

calming 5–7, 75
cancer 109
carpal tunnel syndrome 109–10

case histories
  Jackie Keirs 168–72
  Mr G. 164–8
catarrh see nasal congestion
cerebral palsy 110, 173
Channels,
  energetic quality of 37
  and Internal Organs 39
  and Ki 9–10
  locations of 10–32
  and moxa 162–3
childbirth 110–11
children and Shiatsu 173
chiropractic 103, 106, 118, 120, 151
clothing 1, 76, 79, 82
Cold 68–9
cold, common 111
comfort 81–2
constipation 112–13
constitution, poor 69–70
continuity 86–7
control cycle 60, 65
convalescence 113
coronary artery disease 97–8, 98,
    103
counselling 95, 102, 114, 129, 132,
    145
cramp 113–14
Creation Cycle 60
cross fibre stretching 139, 156
cuts 90

Dampness 69
definition of Shiatsu vii
depression 114
dermatitis 115
diabetes mellitus 115, 128
diagnosis 2, 34–5
  see also assessment, Shiatsu
    health
diarrhoea 116
diet 70, 96, 97, 136
disease 66–71
  external causes of 68–9
  infectious 89, 130
  internal causes of 68–8

other causes of 69–71
dispersal 5, 6, 86
diverticulosis 116
Down's syndrome 117
Dryness 68–9

earache 117–18
Earth 60, 64, 65
eczema 118
effectiveness of Shiatsu, limited 88
elderly and Shiatsu 174
empathy 87
emphysema 118
energy 8–9
environment for Shiatsu 1–2
Essence 40, 44, 45, 47, 63
eye soreness 118

facial palsy 119
fainting 119
fatigue 119–20
fear 66, 67
Feldenkrais method 106
fever 89, 120
fibrositis 120–121
fingertips 2–3
Fire 60, 64, 65
Five Elements 59–66
  and correspondences within
    humans 62, 65–6
flat feet 121
flu see fever
fluency 86–7
fractures 121
frequency of Shiatsu 175
frozen shoulder 121

Gall Bladder, function of 57–8
glandular fever 122–3
golfer's elbow see tennis elbow
gout 103
gravity, low centre of 81
grounding, sense of viii, 144, 159

haemorrhoids 123
harmony, importance of 33

Hay diet 130
hay fever 123
headaches 124
Heart,
    and Blood 41
    and Body Fluids 43
    function of 53–4
    and Mind 46
    and Sense Organs 45
    and Tissues 43
heart attack 124–5
Heart protector, function of 54
Heat 68–9
hemiplegia 93, 125
herbal medicine 69, 95
    passim
hernia 126
herpes 126
hiccups 127
history of Shiatsu ix–x
HIV 95–6, 128
homoeopathy 96, 98, 103
    passim
hormone replacement therapy 131,
    142
Hoshino therapy 91, 99
hyperglycaemia 127
hypochondriasis 128
hypoglycaemia 128

imbalance 8–9, 66, 76
    hormonal 93, 110
immunodeficiency disorders 128
impotence 129
incontinence 129–30
indigestion 130
infections 90
insomnia 131–2
Internal Organs,
    and Blood 41
    and Body Fluids 42–3
    and Channels 39
    functions of 47–58
    and Ki 40–41
    and Mental Faculties 46–7
    and Sense Organs 45

and Tissues 43–4
intestines, twisted 90
irritable bowel syndrome 132

jaundice 97, 122
jet lag 132
Jitsu 37–8
joint injuries 133

Ki 8–9
    circulation of 9–10
    essential qualities of 79–87
    functions of 8–9, 52–3, 56–7
    and health assessment 76
    and Internal Organs 40–41
    and Kidneys 40, 47–8
    and Liver 41, 56–7
    and Lungs 40, 49–50
    and Mind 85
    and moxa 162–3
    and Spleen 40, 50–52
    and Tsubos 35–7
    and Yin/Yang 35
Kidneys,
    and Body Fluids 42–3
    function of 47–8
    and Ki 40, 47–8
    and Sense Organs 45
    and Tissues 44
    and Willpower 47
Kyo 37–8

Large Intestine, function of 50–52
Laws of Cure 160–62
leukorrhoea 133
ligament sprain 90, 134
listening 74
Liver,
    and Blood 41
    and Ethereal Soul 46
    function of 56–7
    and Ki 41, 49–50
    and Sense Organs 45
    and Tissues 43–4
looking 72–3
lordosis 134–5

lumbago *see* backache
Lungs,
    and Body Fluids 42, 50
    and Corporeal Soul 46
    function of 49–50
    and Ki 40
    and Sense Organs 45
    and Tissues 44

M.E. 135–6
massage 99, 140
meditation 70, 80, 156
menopause 136, 142
menstrual disorders 136–7
Metal 60, 65
migraine 137
Mind 9, 46, 80, 82
motivation 80
moxa 116, 162–3
moxibustion 162–3
multiple sclerosis 93, 137–8
muscle stiffness 138–9
muscle strain 90, 140

nasal congestion 140
nausea 141
neurosis 141

occupational therapy 125
osteoarthritis 103
osteopathy 103, 106, 117, 118, 120,
    124, 150, 151, 153
osteoporosis 93, 142
ovarian cyst 142–3
over-exertion 70
overexcitement 67

P.M.T. *see* menstrual disorders
palm heat 90–91, 99, 148
palms 2
palpitations 143
panic attacks 143–4
paralysis 144
paranoia 144–5
phobia 145
physiotherapy 103, 110, 121, 125, 153

piles *see* haemorrhoids
polio 146
positive connection 85–6
pregnancy 90, 146–7
pressure, correctly-angled 86
preventative therapy, Shiatsu as
    174–5
prolapsed uterus 147
prostate problems 147–8
psoriasis 148
psychosis 149
psychotherapy 100, 102, 104, 114,
    128, 129, 143–4

Qi Gong 95–6, 119–20, 127, 144, 156

rapport 85–6
reactions to treatment 83–5, 160–62
recovery, indications of 161–2
reflexology 109–10, 115, 119–20, 130
relaxation 81–2, 143–4
respiratory disorders 149
rheumatoid arthritis 103–4, 109–10
running injuries 149

sacroiliac strain 150
sadness 68
schizophrenia *see* psychosis
sciatica 150–51
scoliosis 151
Sense Organs
    and Heart 45
    and Internal Organs 45
    and Kidneys 45
    and Liver 45
    and Lungs 45
    and Spleen 45
sexual activity, excessive 71
Shiatsu Society 74, 80
shock 67–8, 151–2
shoulder stiffness 152
sinusitis *see* nasal congestion
skin problems 89
slipped disc *see* sciatica
Small Intestine 54–5
sore throat 153

Sotai corrective exercises 99,
129–30, 134, 135, 147, 149, 151,
159, 163
spastic paralysis 153
Spleen,
    and Blood 41, 50–52
    and Body Fluids 42
    function of 50–52
    and Ki 40, 50–52
    and Sense Organs 45
    and thought 47
    and Tissues 44
sports injuries 153
stammering 154
stomach, acid 94
Stomach, function of 52–3
stress 82, 124–5, 131, 136, 138,
154–5
stroke see hemiplegia
support 82–5, 86, 96, 109

Tai Ji Quan viii, 70, 80, 102
technique vii, 3–7, 86–7
tennis elbow 155–6
tension 124, 156
therapist, good vii, 2, 38, 74, 79, 87,
94, 144
thrombosis 156
thumbs 2
tinnitus 157
Tissues,
    and Heart 43
    and Internal Organs 43–4

and Kidneys 44
and Liver 43–4
and Lungs 44
and Spleen 44
tonification 4, 7, 86
tools of Shiatsu 2–3
toothache 157
touch 74–6, 85–6, 89, 91, 155, 175
toxaemia 158
trauma 71
travel sickness 158
treatment,
    reactions to 83–5, 160–62
    receiving 76–9
Triple Heater 47
    function of 55–6
Tsubo 35–7, 75

varicose veins 90, 158–9
vertigo 159

Water 59, 60, 63, 65
whiplash injuries 159
Wind 68
Wood 59–60, 63–4, 65
worry and pensiveness 68

Yin/Yang 33–5, 39, 59, 64, 66, 71
yoga viii, 70, 80, 102, 120, 127, 144,
156

Zangfu Organs 39, 58